"The Many Benefits Of Coconuts, Peanuts, And Other Tasty Nut Foods!"

"The Many Benefits Of Coconuts, Peanuts, And Other Tasty Nut Foods!"

Published By Joseph A. Laydon Jr.

Website: http://www.survivalexpertebooks.com

E-Mail: wwwsurvivalexpert@yahoo.com

MOST IMPORTANT NOTE: The individual *"The Many Benefits Of Coconuts, Peanuts, And Other Tasty Nut Foods!"* is a compilation from my already published Anytime Anywhere Survival Newsletters (Newsletter) at http://www.survivalexpert.com

Published By Joseph A. Laydon Jr.

Website: http://www.survivalexpertebooks.com

E-Mail: wwwsurvivalexpert@yahoo.com

Copyright & Disclaimer

IRISAP DISCLAIMER STATEMENT

The author of *"The Many Benefits Of Coconuts, Peanuts, And Other Tasty Nut Foods"* and owner of Intensive Research Information Services And Product(s) (IRISAP) is exercising his right under the First Amendment to self-publish and co-author this informational product to better educate the public with respect to being more self-reliant Anytime Anywhere. The author is publishing this information based upon his "intensive research" and his experiences. Author is demonstrating through this Special Report how to become self-reliant in survival situations.

This book is designed to help the reader become more aware of the unique benefits of Coconuts and Nut Foods.

The information is for educational purposes only. Professional advice from "qualified "medical professionals " is ALWAYS and HIGHLY recommended. Advice is neither implied nor intended. IRISAP and authors\writers of resource materials are not responsible for the purchaser's and third party activities and is in no way responsible for sickness or death or successes.

THE PURCHASER OF THIS SPECIAL REPORT IS SOLELY RESPONSIBLE FOR THIRD PARTY DISCLOSURE AND RESPONSIBLE FOR THEIR ACTIONS AND ANY PRIVATE OR PROFESSIONAL ACTIONS TAKEN FROM THIS INFORMATIONAL PRODUCT.

This Special Report is Copyrighted and VIOLATORS WILL BE PROSECUTED! If the consumer DISAGREES with ANY portion of this DISCLAIMER STATEMENT, the consumer MUST immediately (upon receipt) return this entire informational product for a full refund.

Table Of Contents

Contents

Dedication!

This book – ***"The Many Benefits Of Coconuts, And Other Tasty Nut Foods!"*** is dedicated to all the past, present and future sickly and dead patients who put their total trust in conventional medicine of drugs and surgery. Conventional Medicine is not the sole answer to a healthy and vibrant life.

There are better alternatives to the multitudes of sickly therapies of drugs used in conventional medicine.

There are more than 60 Alternative Therapies. 60 Alternative Therapies that are worthy of your attention. The 667-page Gettysburg Program found at http://www.survivalexpertbooks.com is where the Gettysburg Program and other data can be found concerning Alternative Therapies used throughout the world and throughout history.

This Book - ***"The Many Benefits Of Coconuts, And Other Tasty Nut Foods!"*** barely, barely, barely touches all those 60+ Alternative Therapies. I highly encourage you to see all my Electronic Books for much more Self-Reliance Data. SEE *More Kindle E-Books And Paperback Books For You* at the end of this book.

And don't forget to see Survival Expert at http://www.survivalexpert.com

Introduction

Coconut palms are grown in more than 90 different countries that have tropical wet climates. Coconuts are even grown in the Unites States in Hawaii and central and southern Florida. And her protected territories like American Samoa, Guam, Puerto Rico, Virgin Islands and the Common Wealth of the Northern Marinna Islands.

According to the United States Food & Drug Administration, the coconut is considered a tree nut.

The coconut palm grows as high as 98-feet high. Its leaves grow up to 20-feet long. It's estimated that **150 people per year are KILLED BY FALLING COCONUTS!** That's 10-times more people killed than by them ornery sharks!

It takes up to 10-years to produce coconuts. A single coconut palm can provide as many as 75 coconuts per year. Total world production of coconuts is approximately 62 million tons per year.

In this book, you'll read about the many uses of the coconut like nourishment, alternative health care practices, first-aid, fire-starting, cosmetics, weight-loss,... and much more interesting information.

Super Benefits Of Coconuts!

The following are several healthy benefits of the coconut and all its parts young or mature. Let's start with the healthy *Benefits Of Coconut Water*.

Benefits Of Coconut Water: Here are several benefits of *Coconut Water* (not coconut milk - found in mature coconuts).

a) Fresh Young Green Coconuts: Once you open a young coconut, the meat must be the color of white snow. If it's pinkish or even the slightest shade of pink - throw it away. However, the water of a fresh young coconut - '*Coconut Water*,' it will have a slight tea color to it. For a good video on young green coconuts, see *How To Open A Coconut In 30 Seconds* on YouTube.

b) Coconut Water: *Coconut Water* comes from the young green coconuts versus the coconut milk that comes from mature coconuts. Young fresh coconuts can be purchased from specialty healthfood stores. You may also put in a request for *"young green coconuts."*

c) Coconut Water: *Coconut Water* helps lower bad cholesterol levels (HDL) that are a risk for heart disease. *Coconut Water* also helps with digestion, improves libido, dissolves kidney stones, and fights bladder and urinary tract infections. An old Philippine saying goes something like '*A coconut a day keeps the urologist away.*'

d) Digestion Aid: *Coconut Water* has more hydrating properties than tap water and may aid in better digestion of foods meaning absorbing more of the nutrients in the food you eat along with drinking *Coconut Water.*

e) Energy Drink Replacement: *Coconut Water* could be your replacement for those expensive energy drinks. *Coconut Water* provides less sodium while providing more potassium. Potassium helps regulate the water balance within the body and transports nutrients. This mineral is also instrumental in helping send messages through our nervous system. The heart and other muscles are dependent on potassium for a healthy state and their proper function.

f) Fluid of Life: Some natives around the world where coconuts are found, call the coconut the *"Fluid of Life."*

g) Hydration: If you're dehydrated whether in a survival situation, athletic sports or after a binge of drinking,... *Coconut Water* may be the quick remedy to quick hydration. Plus you get the nutrition and electrolytes much needed by the dehydrated body. *Coconut Water* can be used to fight-off dehydration by drinking it prior, during and after forecasted events where the body is physically stressed.

h) Blood Replacement: The electrolytes found in *Coconut Water* are about the same levels found in your plasma.

Electrolytes are ionized salts in blood, tissue fluids and cells including salts of sodium and potassium. A substance that can conduct electricity when it is in solution. So? So what? We need electrolytes because our entire body is an electrical system and we need those electrolytes to keep us performing at our best whether we're running in a marathon or sitting behind a desk. In emergency situations, *Coconut Water* can be used as a substitute for blood.

i) Nutritious: *Coconut Water* provides calcium, chloride, magnesium, potassium,... while its low in protein, sodium, sugar,... Plus like I said it's loaded with electrolytes.

j) Other Benefits Of Coconut Water: Researchers out of India found that *Coconut Water* may aid in reducing symptoms of heart disease. Different studies found that *Coconut Water* may help to detoxify the liver. And Coconut Water may aid to lower bad cholesterol (LDL).

k) PMS Cure: This segment comes from Woman's World Magazine, by Amy Capetta (13 February 2007 - [page 26). As a young lady, Katie developed all out PMS in her 20s! Trying every remedy she knew, nothing worked and she was a sickly mess with severe mood swings, fatigue, headaches, cramps, irritable bowel syndrome,... Finally a friend told her to try *Coconut Water*. Katie drank a 12-ounce bottle of *Coconut Water* 03-times a week.

Noticing little changes almost immediately, it was only 03-weeks later she realized she wasn't stricken with severe mood swings, fatigue, headaches, cramps, irritable bowel syndrome,... Now she drinks *Coconut Water* BEFORE and DURING each period. Katie says: *"Thanks to coconut water, all my days are good."*

l) **Virus Fighter**: *Coconut Water* has anti-viral and anti-fungal properties and may help to fight the flu, cold and other common maladies.

m) **Genuine Coconut Water Products**: Genuine *Coconut Water* can be purchased at some healthfood stores. Some name brands that offer a genuine *Coconut Water* are O.N.E., VitaCoco and Zico. Look for *Coconut Water* at your local healthfood store. Now let's carry-on with *NG Trobriand Skinny Diet*.

NG Trobriand Skinny Diet: Since most Americans are overweight, I thought I'd add this diet. In the South Pacific lay the Trobriand Islands and obesity is about non-existent. Why? They eat no fried foods. As a matter of fact their diet is mainly composed of fish, coconuts, and steamed vegetables. It's that simple. (National Geographic - July 1992)

Bacteria Proof: The outer shell of the coconut (young and old) keeps bacteria and parasites away from the liquid and meat of the coconut.

Pacific Cavity Free Teeth: Yapese adults carry a betel-nut basket that is hand-woven. The betel-nut basket holds aged or hollow coconut shell that are filled with lime powder. The lime powder is made from crushed coral. The coconut shell also holds betel nuts and leaves. The betel nut is split open and sprinkled with lime powder. This is wrapped in a leaf and chewed. The betel nut releases a red dye which reddens - stains the teeth and gums and has been used for ages to make their teeth cavity-proof.

Now here's some very healthy data concerning coconut oil and worth 1,000-times the cost of this book - *The Many Healthy Benefits Of Oil Pulling.*

The Many Healthy Benefits Of Oil Pulling: In the year 2000, the Surgeon General of the United States issued a report - *"Oral Health in America,"* noting the unknown unhealthy link between oral health and overall health. The *"Oral Health in America"* Report is the *"silent factor promoting the onset of life-threatening diseases which are responsible for the deaths of millions of Americans each year."*

Your mouth is home to **BILLIONS** of bacteria, viruses, fungi, parasites,… and myriad other toxins. And strains of germs such as candida and streptococcus and their toxic waste products not only cause gum disease and tooth decay, but also contribute to serious and even debilitating health problems.

With the billions of bacteria, viruses, fungi, parasites,… and myriad other toxins in your mouth, your immune system is overburdened by factors such as excessive stress, poor diet, and environmental toxins, destructive organisms from your mouth can spread throughout the body. Once unleashed in the body, these toxins can generate secondary infections, chronic inflammation, and other persistent health problems.

The Mayo Clinic (Jacksonville, Florida -USA) staff lists the following diseases and conditions that may be caused or affected by oral health:
• Cardiovascular disease
• Endocarditis (infection of the inner lining of the heart)
• Premature birth and low birth weight
• Diabetes
• HIV/AIDS
• Eating disorders
• Osteoporosis
• Alzheimer's disease
• Immune system disorders

In 2013, I started reading at what is called Oil Pulling. Oil Pulling is simply swishing a few teaspoons of oil (coconut oil) in your mouth for 30-minutes each day. The 30-minutes of swishing the oil around in your mouth and then spitting it all out has a list of benefits. Back in April 2014, I tried Oil Pulling just 03-times, only 03-times for only 20-mintes each time and I got immediate relief from nasal congestion and bleeding gums.

That was my brief R & D. Now here's a list of the benefits of Oil Pulling:

- Arthritis
- Asthma
- Bad Breath
- Bleeding Gums
- Body Detox
- Boosts Immune System
- Clearer Mind
- Congestion
- Decreased Joint Pain
- Elimination Of Allergies
- Enhances Kidney Function
- Enhances Liver Function
- Gum Disease
- Gums Restored To Pink Color
- Hangover
- Headaches
- Improves Acne
- Improved Cardiovascular
- Improved Sleep
- Improves Skin Condition
- Increased Energy
- Increased Metabolism
- Jaw Soreness
- Migraines
- Nasal / Sinus Congestion
- TMJ

- Tooth Decay
- Vision Improvement
- Whiter Teeth

MOST IMPORTANT NOTE: After putting this segment together, I am convinced of the benefits of Oil Pulling and will start a schedule immediately.

Oil Pulling is used with sunflower oil, olive oil, or **<u>coconut oil</u>**. Most prefer coconut oil. Why? Cause coconut oil has Anti-Bacteria, Anti-Fungal, and Anti-Viral properties which gives your own immune system a better chance to improve your health cause now it can fight other bad guys throughout your body.

Coconut Oil: Here's a quote from my book the *Gettysburg Program* (full version) concerning healthy coconut oil: Coconut oil got a bad rap years ago. Sixty-five percent of coconut oil's saturated fat is mostly made up of medium-chain triglycerides (MCTs). Populations like Polynesian Puka Puka and Tokelau islanders that consume most of their fat from coconut oil have **<u>low rates of heart disease!</u>**

Coconut oil, unlike other oils, is less likely to attribute to obesity. Why? Your body easily converts coconut oil into energy rather than depositing calories as body fat.

Coconut oil also kills germs! It contains anti-microbial components like mother's milk. The Polynesian Puku Puku and Tokelau islanders live in an environment ideal for parasites. There protected from parasites by the coconut oil in their diet.

It may be wise to avoid processed products like margarine, chips, cookies... that have trans-fatty acids. According to a study Dr. Walter Willett, of Harvard University, trans-fatty acids double the risk of heart attack. Trans-fatty acids may also contribute to cancer, diabetes and obesity. Read the contents before you purchase the product. Look for *"partially hydrogenated oils."* If you read this, AVOID IT!

The fresh white coconut meat is protein rich and loaded with coconut oil. Coconut oil is rich in what is called lauric acid which is found in Mother's milk. Lauric acid has anti-bacteria, anti-fungal, and anti-viral agents. The super healthy fresh coconut oil and fresh white meat have a laundry list of super healthy benefits like:
- Anti-Bacteria
- Anti-Fungal
- Anti-Viral
- Candida Albicans
- Chronic Fatigue
- Chron's Disease
- Diabetes
- Digestive Disorders
- Energy Booster

- Heart Disease
- IBS (irritable bowel syndrome
- Immune System Booster
- Lowers Cholesterol
- Metabolism Booster
- Rejuvenate Skin
- Thyroid Function
- Weight-Loss
- Wrinkles

Pacific Coconut Parts!

Here are some coconut parts and their uses by Pacific Islanders. OK, let's start with coconut roots:

a) Roots: Roots were used to make medicine and used as a fertilizer.

b) Trunk: The trunk of the coconut tree is durable and hard wood to make furniture, used for many construction projects, used to make bridges (Bridge Over The River Kwai?).

c) Bark: The bark (towards the top of the tree) of the coconut tree is used to make strainers, rags, clothing, sandals,...

d) Blossom Sheath: The blossom sheath (tops of tree where young coconut nuts emerge) is used for firewood, used for funnels, toys,...

e) Blossom: The blossom is tapped for tuba. Tuba is a white coconut sap. Tuba can be prepared and used a few ways like a sweetener, alcoholic beverage, vinegar or a syrup.

f) Nut Stems: The nut stems are used for decoration, firewood, fertilizer,...

g) Baby Nut: The young baby nut can be used for food, toys,...

h) Immature Nut: The young coconut nut's husk is used to make rope, to buff, wipe, sponge, toilet paper, fertilizer,... It's burned to produce a smudge to repel mosquitoes. It can be carved to make flatware,...

i) Young Shell: The young shell is young enough, can be eaten.

j) Mature Coconut: The hard shell can be carved to make various tools, weapons, flatware,... The 02 empty halves can be used as a bra. The hard shell is a great kindling.

k) Coconut Meat: The coconut meat is used to make a sauce, candy, soap, coconut oil,...

Note: Nowhere have I found evidence of coconut meat being used as kindling.

l) Leaf: The durable leaves are used for paddles, stirring utensil,...

m) Ribs: The ribs of the coconut leaves - namely the stems, are used to make toothpicks for dental hygiene, make brooms,...

n) Frond: The thinner leaves of the coconut tree are called fronds and are used for weaving to make baskets, fans, hats, mats,... You must see the 2003 & 2004 Newsletters for my Coconut R&D.

o) Milk: The coconut milk is a very beneficial drink.

Coconut Personal Care & First-Aid Products!

Coconut Oil and other coconut ingredients are so beneficial, that there are multitudes of personal care products and first-aid products out there on the market that have coconut-type ingredients. Here's a partial of these *Personal Care & First-Aid Products*:

Archipelago Coconut Lotion

Bon Vital Coconut Massage Creme

Coconut Oil Hair Shine?

Delon Coconut Oil Body Cream

Dogzymes Ultimate Skin and Coat with Algal Oil and Organic Coconut

Dominican Natural Coconut Oil Skin & Body Care

Eminence Coconut Cream Masque

Face Cream By Mee Beauty

Hugo Naturals Shampoo Smoothing And Defining Coconut

iOrgani Coconut Oil for Hair, Skin and Body

InstaNatural Argan Oil Hair Treatment

Marc Anthony True Professional Hand Cream, Hydrating Coconut Oil & Shea Butter

Mason Natural Coconut Oil Beauty Cream

Mountain Ocean Skin Trip Moisturizer, Coconut

Natures Greatest Secret - Amber Formula - Antibacterial, Antifungal

NOW Solutions - Coconut Oil Skin & Hair Revitalizing

OGX Weightless Hydration Oil, Coconut Water

Palmer's Coconut Oil Formula Curl Condition Hair Pudding

Palmer's Coconut Oil Formula Curl Conditioning Shampoo

Palmer's Coconut Oil Formula Hair Conditioner

Philosophy Coconut Frosting 3-in-1 Shampoo, Body Wash, and Bubble Bath

PurO3 Organic Ozonated Coconut Oil

Puritan's Pride Premium Coconut Oil Skin & Hair Nutrients

RMS Beauty Raw Coconut Cream

Softee Coconut Oil Hair & Scalp Conditioner

Spectrum Essentials Unrefined Organic Coconut Oil Bodycare

I Went Down For The Count!

In 1982 while assigned to the A Co. 3rd Bn. 5th Special Forces Group out of Fort Bragg NC, our team was training in the hilly - mountainous terrain Utah. For several days prior to deployment, I was preparing for this training except for one area - I failed to maintain myself on a high energy diet. Arriving in Utah, I was weak but I didn't complain nor remedy my weakened state.

Pulling point man and patrolling throughout the Utah hilly terrain, the hard rocky terrain, cold weather, snow, and my heavy pack were taking its toll on my already low energy and weak body.

After several hours negotiating the steep terrain, my legs collapsed from underneath me and down I went but I couldn't get up. My team members came to my aid wondering what was wrong with me. Answering the very well-trained savvy medic's rapid questions he concluded I was only mal-nourished and needed food. I told them I hadn't eaten right for several days preparing for this deployment - I was too busy to eat a full meal.

The medic and the commo man laughingly called me a *"dumb ass"* repeatedly while the Team Sergeant pulled out 01 of 02 full bags of trail-mix from his rucksack. He gave me a full heavy bag of trail-mix and ordered me to eat it as I lay there on my back. I ate greedily and was rejuvenated almost immediately and boy was that trail-mix GOOD!

It had several kinds of nuts (fatty oils), raisins, check's cereal squares, chocolate pieces, **coconut slices**, dried banana slices, dried fig slices, dried peach slices, and several other nutritious ingredients. The Team Sergeant had his own concoction and after that memorable incident I started carrying my own trail-mix. It's a quick energizing fuel. So remember my memorable lesson and consider carrying a bag of quick-energy trail-mix on your next outdoor adventure. And don't forget to add some high energy pinon nuts to the trail-mix concoction. See *Kjoules Table - Energy Ratings For Nuts* at the end of this book.

Laydon's Survival Trail-Mix!

Let's carry-on with a trail-mix with hand-picked ingredients that I've come up with that are loaded with FUEL THAT WILL PHYSICALLY AND MENTALLY ENERGIZE YOU so you're ready Anytime Anywhere and I call it *Laydon's Survival Trail-Mix*. No, I'm not into myself, it's a protective copyright thing - it's a *"writer's thing"* - besides it's my book and I can do what I want - especially when it helps you out so you're ready Anytime Anywhere!

Here are all the ingredients to *Laydon's Survival Trail-Mix*:

- Almond M&Ms
- Milk Chocolate M&Ms Candies
- Banana Slices
- Brazil Nuts
- Chocolate Raisins
- **Coconut Slices or Flakes**
- Corn Nuts
- Honey Roasted Peanuts
- Honey
- Pineapple Slices
- Pinon Nuts
- Soybean Nuts
- Pumpkin Seeds

OK, now let me tell you about the nutritious details of each of these tasty ingredients. Let's start with Almond M&Ms.

a) Almond M&Ms: Almond M&Ms provide the nutritious almond nut and tasty chocolate. First let's cover the benefits of the almond nut then we'll cover the benefits of tasty chocolate.

The almond is cultivated in the United States and its reddish hardwood is used by cabinetmakers. But it's delicious nuts are harvested for food. The almond nut itself contains a nutritious bland oil, emulsin, gum and mucilage sugar that have agreeable sweet tastes. The chocolate coating just adds more flavor and complimented with the several side benefits of eating chocolate.

According to USDA (United States Department of Agriculture - James Penland Ph.D.) research, found that trail-mix is full of boron which BOOSTS mental alertness by 10%! Those subjects with low levels of boron had 'sluggish brains.' And eating trail-mix corrects the boron deficiency almost instantly. Boron comes in trail-mix foods like raisins, almonds, peanuts, hazelnuts,...

b) Milk Chocolate M&Ms Candies: Milk chocolate M&Ms candies were first made in 1941 and the original colors were brown, green, red, violet, & yellow and were packaged in a paper tube. Chocolate M&Ms are known around the world and as far back as WWII. According to the booklet The World Of M&M/MARS, "When the United States entered World War II, M&Ms soon became a success as part of the U.S service personnel rations." See Chocolate in the A-Z Index.

c) Banana Slices: A medium bananas furnishes only 100 calories, has hardly any sodium and is a modest source of Vitamin C. Bananas also furnish fiber for the heart healthy concerned and provides potassium which helps controlling blood pressure. Bananas are packed with Vitamin B6 which helps prevent depression. One banana provides 35% of the B6 RDA. Eating a banana helps combat hunger pangs and leaves you feeling satisfied and full. Bananas also help you remain alert and energetic because of the fructose sugar that is encased in fiber and carbohydrates is slowly released into your system.

In the 1930s, medical literature noted that bananas were a cure for ulcers. Experimenting with mice, researchers isolated a chemical in ripe and unripe bananas that suppressed acid secretion, thus blocking the development of ulcers in animals.

Modern teams of British and Indian researchers have discovered why the banana-eating rodents end up with about 1/3 fewer and less severe ulcers. Bananas work just like the most sophisticated drugs (carbenoxolone), but without the side-effects like high blood pressure. Bananas strengthen the surface cells of the stomach lining, forming a sturdier barrier against noxious juices. The British researchers' bottom line: *"The role of bananas in folk medicine as an antiulcerogenic agent, at least against gastric ulcers, appears justified...."* See *Laydon Family Remedy That Cures Ulcer & Other Intestinal Problems* in the December 2001 Newsletter.

d) Brazil Nuts: Brazil Nut Tree (Bertholletia excelsa), native to northern Brazil is the common name for a tropical tree that reaches a height of approximately 100-feet high. The tree produces a round, woody seed vessel, about the size of a grapefruit, which contains as many as 24 triangular Brazil nuts.

The triangular nut has a hard brown rough-surfaced shell that encloses an oily white kernel that's the size of an adult thumb. Brazil nuts are loaded with nutrients to include oil for fuel for your body and fire-starting fuel. An average Brazil kernel burns for a whopping 06-minutes and 30-seconds; plenty - plenty of time to get a life-saving fire going.

Brazil Nuts are rich in selenium which is an antioxidant linked to low rates of cancer and heart disease. According to Donald J. Lisk at Cornell University, just eating one Brazil nut a day would keep you sufficient in selenium. However, eating more than one-half dozen Brazil nuts everyday could cause nausea to some folks.

Brazil nuts are gluten free (wheat allergies, Celiac Disease,…), and also provide Vitamin E (antioxidant), B vitamins (folate, niacin, pantothenic acid, pyridoxine, and riboflavin), calcium, copper, iron, manganese, magnesium, phosphorus, potassium, and zinc.

The Brazil nut also provide needed amino acids, namely arginine cysteine, glutamine, glutamic acid, linoleic, oleic, palmitic, and alpha linolenic acids. The role of amino acids are for the manufacture of protein and muscle.

e) Chocolate Raisins: If you don't know it by now, raisins are nothing more than dried-up grapes. Raisins are Mother Nature's tasty candy and when dried from grapes to raisins they're concentrated natural candies of nutrition. Besides their sweet taste, raisins provide a bounty of **Vitamin B1 (THIAMINE). Vitamin B1 enhances circulation and assists in the production of hydrochloric acid, blood formation and carbohydrate formation.

Vitamin B1 affects energy, growth disorders and learning capacity. Vitamin B1 is needed for muscle tone of the intestines, stomach and heart. Thiamin is noted as a brain booster because it helps produce the messages your brain sends out to nerve cells. Thiamin is vital to memory and learning. Sources of Vitamin B1 are asparagus, broccoli, Brussels sprouts, dried beans, brown rice, egg yolks, fish, organ meats (kidney, liver, heart), many nuts, oatmeal, peanuts, peas, plums, pork, poultry, dried prunes, raisins, rice bran, sardines, soybeans, turkey, wheat germ and whole grain.

Raisins also provide boron. According to USDA (United States Department of Agriculture - James Penland Ph.D.) research, found that trail-mix is full of boron which BOOSTS mental alertness by 10%!

Those subjects with low levels of boron had 'sluggish brains.' And eating trail-mix corrects the boron deficiency almost instantly. Boron comes in trail-mix foods like raisins, almonds, peanuts, hazelnuts,...

f) Coconut Slices: I gave you a lot of survival data and my own copyrighted R&D on life-saving coconuts in the 2003 and 2004 Newsletters. Before you carry-on with this segment, you ought to return to those Newsletters and get reacquainted with that survival data. I'll wait right here till you get back,....

OK, you're back. Here's some super healthy data on coconuts and why you should not only take fresh coconuts on all your outdoor adventures but also have coconut slices in your trail-mix.
According to Cookycoconuts.com, nutritional values change as the coconut matures. Move aside Gatorade - for the liquid inside the coconut is coconut water or called coconut juice and is one of the HIGHEST sources of electrolytes on Earth. Electrolytes are ionized salts in blood, tissue fluids and cells including salts of sodium and potassium. A substance that can conduct electricity when it is in solution. So? So what? We need electrolytes because our entire body is an electrical system and we need those electrolytes to keep us performing at our best whether we're running in a marathon or sitting behind a desk.

And the coconut juice is consumed to prevent dehydration, and is used in some areas of the world to hydrate casualties via intravenous tubes and needles.

The fresh white coconut meat is protein rich and loaded with coconut oil. Coconut oil is rich in what is called lauric acid which is found in Mother's milk. Lauric acid has anti-bacteria, anti-fungal, and anti-viral agents. The super healthy fresh coconut oil and fresh white meat have a laundry list of super healthy benefits like:

- Anti-Bacteria
- Anti-Fungal
- Anti-Viral
- Candida Albicans
- Chronic Fatigue
- Chron's Disease
- Diabetes
- Digestive Disorders
- Energy Booster
- Heart Disease
- IBS (irritable bowel syndrome
- Immune System Booster
- Lowers Cholesterol
- Metabolism Booster
- Rejuvenate Skin
- Thyroid Function
- Weight-Loss
- Wrinkles

Bottom line, now you know plenty of good reasons to mix plenty of fresh coconut slices in your trial-mix.

1st Note: http://www.cookycoconuts.com recommends the best brand coconut oil is Tropical Traditions. See Tropical Traditions in the POC Section.

And for more weight-loss data, see SPECIAL Intelligence Report #309 - <u>"149+ Lose It Or Else Accelerated Weight-Loss Facts & Tricks!"</u>

2nd Note: You must see *Coconut Kindling*. Today (02 May 2005), I took the same bag of old coconut slices (19 May 2003) that are almost 02-years old and ate a slice. Stale yes, but that small old coconut slice still fired-up with all its spitting fireworks like it was a fresh slice. See *Lost Coconut R&D* (fire-starting).

3rd Note: I know what you're asking. Does a fresh dripping wet piece of fresh coconut still fire-up? You're darn right it does. Just concentrate your match on specific spot on a thin piece of coconut (I used a thick piece) and it will fire-up. Why? Cause even though the coconut is wet from its coconut milk, it will still fire-up because of the piece of coconut is loaded with fuel - coconut oil. However, to make sure it fires-up real quick, I'd lay plenty of thin slices of fresh coconut out in the open dry air so to rid them of the coconut water.

g) Corn Nuts: Them tasty corn nuts provide plenty of nutrition. A 06-ounce package of Sunny Orchard Corn Nuts contains 12 grams of fat, 1,080 milligrams of sodium, a whopping 132 grams of carbohydrates, 06 grams of fiber, and 18 grams of protein. Sunny Orchard may contain trace elements of Vitamins A & C, calcium, and iron.

h) Honey Roasted Peanuts: Regular ol' peanuts are so beneficial, I had to give a large direct quote from the April 2003 Newsletter and here it is in its entirety (is this a word?). Again the following *"peanut"* article is taken directly from the April 2003 Newsletter.

Peanuts are nutritious and high in energy. The seeds contain 40 to 50 percent oil and 20 to 30 percent protein, and an excellent source of B Vitamins. About half the peanuts grown in the United States are made into peanut butter, and one-fourth are sold as roasted peanuts. Peanut oil is also popular as a high-quality salad and cooking oil and is commonly used in margarine. In the United States peanuts are grown primarily for food; in other countries they are used principally for edible oil. See *14 Peanut Butter Facts!*

Now at the beginning of this segment, I stated *"honey roasted peanuts."* Why? Well if you got peanuts why not make them honey roasted cause that honey is a natural nutritious substance that will also help you physically and mentally Anytime Anywhere. Now let's talk a bit about the *"food fit for the gods"* - honey. See *14 Peanut Butter Facts* below.

i) Honey: **Greeks regarded it as *"food fit for the gods!"* Besides being extremely tasty, honey is noted to be easy on the digestive system because the bees have already digested it.

It's acts as an antiseptic and helps relieve burns, skin abrasions and even bee stings! Honey provides many nutrients like calcium, copper, iron, manganese, magnesium, phosphorus, potassium, silica, sodium and Vitamin C from pollen. AVOID honey in your local grocery store, because it is heat treated and filtered. Purchase honey at health food stores. Insure it is pure, untreated and unfiltered honey (cloudy with healthful pollen). Your best bet is to go out in the countryside and look for honey farmers. INSURE you ask them if pesticides are used on any part of their land or neighboring farm lands. If so, the pesticides may be passed on to the honey.

Important Note: Here are honey's super nutritious and health-enhancing cousins you have to know about. Let's start with Bee Pollen.

1) **Bee Pollen**: Did you know honey bee pollen is one of the world's oldest health foods for the athlete? Bee Pollen is a very fine powder making up the male element of flower. Those busy bees gather pollen in microscopic amounts and carry it to their hive. Bees instinctively collect the most nutritious and healthy bee pollen.

Bee Pollen provides amino acids, calcium, carotene, copper, enzymes, iron, magnesium, manganese, polyunsaturated fatty acids, potassium, sodium, plant sterols, simple sugars, B-Complex and Vitamin C. Bee Pollen combats cancer, colon disorders, depression and fatigue. Honey is noted for its antiseptic and salve for burns.

Many experts have stated that honey bee pollen is nature's most perfect food. Alin Callas, a French agriculturist, studied the question of honey bee pollen being nature's most perfect food and he concluded that a person could literally live on 35 grams of bee pollen per day, satisfying all of the human body's nutritional requirements! Alin Callas said 20 grams of honey bee pollen could be used as a survival diet if need be.

Bonny Laboratories of Geneva, Switzerland discovered that honey bee pollen contains total nutrition!
* Protein = 35%.
* Carbohydrates = 40%.
* Fat = 5%.
* Minerals (27) and carrier molecules and other unidentified ingredients = 3%.

* Moisture = 3-4%.
* Vitamins, trace elements, B Complex Vitamins, Vitamins A, C, D & E and natural antibiotics = 13%-14%.

Dr. Nicolae Tsitsin, of the Longevity Institute of (then) U.S.S.R., studied 150 of 200 people in Russia living past the age 100 years. He discovered that the majority of these people were beekeepers that ate scrap honey loaded with honey bee pollen!

During the 1976 Olympics, Finnish track coach Antti Lananaki attributed the success of his Olympic athletes to honey bee pollen. One Finnish athlete who won the 5,000 and 10,000 meter races in 1972 and 1976 claimed that his daily intake of honey bee pollen (06-8 tablets) was instrumental to his superior athletic performance. Other success stories come from athletes in the United States, Great Britain...

2) **Propolis:** Propolis comes from the Greek word meaning *"defense before a town."* Propolis is a resinous substance that is gathered and metabolized by those busy bees. It's gathered from bark or leaf buds from shedding trees.

Propolis offers amino acids, balsam, caffeic esters, etheric oils, flavonoids, minerals, pollen, resins, Vitamins and wax. Bees compared to most insects and animal are free of bacteria!

An average bee hive has a population of 50,000 to 65,000 bees, is less than 02 cubic feet and has a mean temperature of 95 degrees with a moisture content of 90 percent. An almost perfect environment for bacteria, infection and disease! Yet, it's a super clean environment! Why? The answer is propolis! Propolis offers flavonoids found to be 500 times the potency and healing power of oranges!

WARNING: .05% of the U.S. population is allergic to Bee Pollen. Insure you are not allergic to Bee Pollen prior to using it.

Follow the recommended dosage and instructions from the label and as per your doctor's instructions.

3) **Royal Jelly: Royal Jelly like bee pollen is packed with nutrients. Royal Jelly is the food that is fed ONLY to the Queen Bee in each hive! Royal Jelly is noted to increase the lifespan of the Queen bee 40 times longer than the average worker bee! Royal Jelly is noted to have a nutritious supply of 20 amino acids, minerals, Vitamins and RNA-DNA factors. It's also known for its antibiotic effect. Nutrition Warehouse and BioEnergy Nutrients in the POC Section are just a couple of the companies that offer this nutritious food as well as bee pollen.

WARNING: .05% of the U.S. population is allergic to Bee Pollen. Insure you are not allergic to Bee Pollen prior to using it.

Follow the recommended dosage and instructions from the label and as per your doctor's instructions.

Powerful Bee Pollen, Royal Jelly And Propolis Combination!

How would you like the SUPER COMBINATION of Bee Pollen, Royal Jelly and Propolis all in one tablet form? See your local healthfood store for this super healthy product of your choice.

Wait, I'm not done yet. A radio infomercial I've been monitoring may be worthy of your attention and they offer a super potent bee pollen product called Nature's Potentiated Bee Pollen.

They claim their product is natural of course and especially free of chemicals because the bee pollen is harvested in New Zealand which is noted to be far more chemically free and pollution free than the United States. But here's the secret to Nature's Potentiated Bee Pollen besides it being harvested in a clean environment, it's specially processed so to provide super potency for your body, namely support of your immune system. See Nature's Potentiated Bee Pollen in the POC Section now. OK, let's carry-on with them tasty and nutritious pineapple slices.

j) Pineapple Slices: Two slices of pineapple provide only 90 calories, Vitamin C and very little sodium. When picking fresh pineapples at the supermarket, insure the leaves are dark green. A natural enzyme found in pineapples called bromelain is a nutrient that increases the body's ability to break down fats and protein promoting body metabolism! Pineapple is rich in manganese and helps satisfy your sweet tooth!

k) Pinon Nuts: Also called Pine Nuts. In my November 2000 Newsletter I told you about those fat-rich pinyon nuts! Here's a quote from that Newsletter: *"As a matter of fact 1-pound of pinon nuts contains a whopping 3,000 calories! Pinyon nuts are found in the western United States (Colorado and westward) at elevations of between 4,000 to 7,500 feet. And they're easy to get - just pick em' up off the ground by the handful during the fall and early winter!*

Different tribes of American Indians gathered the calorie-rich nut. And some tribes like the Navajos traded the fat-rich pinyon nuts for much needed supplies from distant Indian tribes to the east that had no access to them. Pinyon nuts (white in color and almost the size of a kernel of corn), could be eaten as they are or roasted so they last a long time like during the winter months."

In my humble opinion, pinon nuts are nutritious life-savers that may have saved the Donner Party - namely one of the Donner Party members that eventually reached help so to alert others that members of the Donner Party were still alive in their isolated freezing white trap of deep snow.

"The Forlorn Hope weakly continued on. They were so weak, to just step over a downed log, they had to roll over it! The last few days they came across a few Indian tribes and they didn't care if they were hostile or not. Some tribes felt pity for the ragged group and did in fact help them with navigation, and food (raw acorns, prepared acorn meal loafs - November 2000 Newsletter). On 17 January, the chief of one Indian village gave Eddy a handful of pine nuts! After eating them, Eddy "felt wonderfully refreshed!"

Let's pause again. In your November 2000 Newsletter I told you about those rat-rich pinyon nuts! Here's a quote from that Newsletter: *"As a matter of fact 01-pound of pinon nuts contains a whopping 3,000 calories!*

Pinyon nuts are found in the western United States (Colorado and westward) at elevations of between 4,000 to 7,500 feet. And they're easy to get - just pick em' up off the ground by the handful during the fall and early winter! Different tribes of American Indians gathered the calorie-rich nut. And some tribes like the Navajos traded the fat-rich pinyon nuts for much needed supplies from distant Indian tribes to the east that had no access to them. Pinyon nuts (white in color and almost the size of a kernel of corn), could be eaten as they are or roasted so they last a long time like during the winter months."

Those pine nuts probably saved everyone's life for Eddy had a new strength. Foster and the 05 women couldn't go any further. They stopped dead in their tracks and Eddy went on! And make sure you read the survival tricks (gathering pine nuts) by the Choinumne Indians coming soon in your April 2001 Newsletter!

17 January 1847, at about an hour before sundown, in the Sacramento Valley, William Eddy being aided by one then two Indians reached Johnson's Ranch of several make-shift cabins where the Ritchie's cabin was located. The others were several miles (06-10) up the trail. Immediately Eddy was put in a bed and cared for while 04 riders set-off with the 2 Indians following Eddy's blood trail to find the other 06 up the trail. The other 06 were found about midnight that night and were finally brought to the settlement on the night of 18 January.

Other riders set-off to spread the word that the Donner Party were still alive! The Forlorn Hope accomplished their mission! Of the 15 that started their trek to find help on 15 December 1846 only 02 men and 05 women survived their trek to find help.

Maybe pine trees as well as peanuts can be grown in many parts of Africa and help curve the high levels of starvation in that part of the world.

According to USDA (United States Department of Agriculture - James Penland Ph.D.) research, found that trail-mix is full of boron which BOOSTS mental alertness by 10%!

Those subjects with low levels of boron had 'sluggish brains.' And eating trail-mix corrects the boron deficiency almost instantly. Boron comes in trail-mix foods like raisins, almonds, peanuts, hazelnuts,...

**Vitamin B1 (THIAMINE). Vitamin B1 enhances circulation and assists in the production of hydrochloric acid, blood formation and carbohydrate formation. Vitamin B1 affects energy, growth disorders and learning capacity. Vitamin B1 is needed for muscle tone of the intestines, stomach and heart. Thiamin is noted as a brain booster because it helps produce the messages your brain sends out to nerve cells. Thiamin is vital to memory and learning. Sources of Vitamin B1 are asparagus, broccoli, Brussels sprouts, dried beans, brown rice, egg yolks, fish, organ meats (kidney, liver, heart), many nuts, oatmeal, peanuts, peas, plums, pork, poultry, dried prunes, raisins, rice bran, sardines, soybeans, turkey, wheat germ and whole grain.

1) Soybean Nuts: Everyone has already heard about the soybean craze going around the country the last few years and I added soybeans in the Laydon Trail-Mix. Why? First let me give you some background information on soybeans and then we'll go into their nutritional content and I'll give you a healthy healing testimonial from a user of soy products. OK, let's get started. Also called soy and soya bean, it's a common name for annual leguminous plant and its seeds (family Leguminosae). The soybean may have originated in eastern China.

The soybean, an ancient food crop in China, Japan, and Korea, was introduced into the United States in the early 1800s. Back then it was grown as a minor forage crop for many years. The development of a soybean-processing industry in the early 1920s propelled soybean cultivation and today the soybean is a leading crop in the United States, behind the huge ranking crops of corn and wheat. The United States produces about 60 percent of the world's soybeans, compared to 14 percent produced by Brazil, 10 percent by China, and lesser percentages by Argentina, Taiwan, Canada, and India. Production in the United States is located chiefly in the Midwest and the lower Mississippi Valley; more than 30 percent of the United States production is exported.

Soybeans are widely cultivated as a farm crop. At
maturity in approximately 100 to 150 days after
planting, depending on variety, location, and weather,
the leaves turn yellow and drop off, and the pods
rapidly become brown and dry. The soybean seeds,
almost spherical in shape, are usually light yellow,
but some rare varieties are black, brown, or green in
color. The soybean seeds have a black, brown, or
yellow hilum (seed scar) and contain about 20 percent
oil and 40 percent protein. In the United States,
soybeans are grown as a row crop and are planted in May
or June, and harvested in the Fall.

The two basic products of the soybean are protein meal
and oil. In the United States, more than 90 percent of
the oil is consumed as margarine, shortening,
mayonnaise, salad oils, and other edible products. The
remains are used in industrial products such as paint,
varnish, linoleum, and rubber fabrics. Soybean meal is
the major source of the protein supplement used in
livestock feeds, which utilize 98 percent of the total
meal produced. Soybean meal is finding increasing use
in human food products in protein-short areas of the
world and elsewhere. Again, the 02 main ingredients of
soybeans are protein meal and oil.

Now here's that true testimonial from a St. Louis
Security Officer that uses soy products. He told me
that after consuming soy products for about 02-months,
he started re-growing hair on his head he lost years
ago. He has renewed vitality and he's more limber
instead of being stiff all the time.

He stated he feels like he's in his 30s instead of his 60s. And there are all kinds of soy products like: chocolate soy milk, soy cookies, soy peanut butter (peanut free), soy nuts, white soy milk,...

**Vitamin B1 (THIAMINE). Vitamin B1 enhances circulation and assists in the production of hydrochloric acid, blood formation and carbohydrate formation. Vitamin B1 affects energy, growth disorders and learning capacity. Vitamin B1 is needed for muscle tone of the intestines, stomach and heart.

Thiamin is noted as a brain booster because it helps produce the messages your brain sends out to nerve cells. Thiamin is vital to memory and learning. Sources of Vitamin B1 are asparagus, broccoli, Brussels sprouts, dried beans, brown rice, egg yolks, fish, organ meats (kidney, liver, heart), many nuts, oatmeal, peanuts, peas, plums, pork, poultry, dried prunes, raisins, rice bran, sardines, soybeans, turkey, wheat germ and whole grain.

m) Pumpkin Seeds: Pumpkin seeds (no shell) provide vital minerals like copper, iron, magnesium, potassium, and zinc. Pumpkin seeds also provide Vitamin E, (beta-carotene) and L-tryptophan which aids in sleeping. Pumpkin seeds also provide L-tryosine which aids to raise the serotonin levels in the brain - thus improving our attitude.

The Zuni Indians roasted pumpkin seeds as a tasty medicinal aid to remedy intestinal disorders like roundworm (living parasites in humans) and tapeworm (intestinal parasite). And pumpkin seeds have long been known to promote prostate health in adult men.

Researchers in Thailand found that eating just 01 to 03 pumpkin seeds a day may help prevent common kidney stones.

Now you have the hand-picked ingredients of Laydon's Survival Trail-Mix and the several specific reasons WHY I chose each ingredient. Heck, if you had to, you could live off this trail-mix.

All you need is a nearby babbling brook of fresh pure water. Bottom line, you have the synergistic ingredients (better together than alone) of the Laydon's Survival Trail-Mix which are: Almond M&Ms, Milk Chocolate M&Ms, Banana Slices, Brazil Nuts, Chocolate Raisins, Coconut Slices, Corn Nuts, Honey Roasted Peanuts, Pineapple Slices, Pinon Nuts, Soybean Nuts, and Pumpkin Seeds. Go to your local grocery store today and make your own batch - I already have - MMMmmmmmm!!

Banana Recipe: Again, the main staple were bananas. To prepare bananas, they cut-off the stem, sliced the banana peel & all into rings an inch thick and rinsed them thoroughly.

If using green bananas, the thorough washing took away much of their bitterness. Anyway, the banana rings were boiled with meat in **coconut milk**. The result was a meal tasting like sweet potatoes!

See *Kjoules Table - Energy Ratings For Nuts* in this book.

14 Peanut Butter Facts!

OK, here are the real facts on super nutritious tasty peanut butter.

Fact 01: American consume approximately 700,000,000 pounds of peanut butter each year! That's about a katrillion zillion peanuts!

Fact 02: Just 02 tablespoons of peanut butter contain 16 grams of fat - the GOOD fat!

Fact 03: Only 02 tablespoons of peanut butter contain 190 calories!

Fact 04: Just 02 tablespoons of peanut butter contain sufficient amounts of folate as 05 raw carrots or 01 1/2 cups of raspberries.

Fact 05: Barely 02 tablespoons of peanut butter contain sufficient amounts of Vitamin E as in 20 apricots or 20 bananas or 20 slices of whole wheat bread!

Fact 06: Only 02 tablespoons of peanut butter contain sufficient amounts of zinc as in 03 cups of cooked broccoli or 40 dried plums.

Fact 07: Just 02 tablespoons of peanut butter contain sufficient amounts of magnesium as 04 cups of cooked pasta or 20 cooked eggs.

Fact 08: Just 02 tablespoons of peanut butter contain sufficient amounts of potassium as in 02 cups of cottage cheese or 1 1/2 cups of blackberries.

Fact 09: Barely 02 tablespoons of peanut butter contain sufficient amounts of copper as in 03 cups of cooked white rice or 06 cups of apple juice.

Fact 10: Only 02 tablespoons of peanut butter contain sufficient amounts of fiber, vitamins, and minerals.

Fact 11: Experts state women can have 04 tablespoons of peanut butter a day while men can go crazy and eat 06 tablespoons of peanut butter a day to cover the RDA (Recommended Daily Allowance)! Look at all that food you have to eat to get the nutrients your body needs whereas all it takes is 04 to 06 tablespoons of peanut butter a day. Plus - MMMmmmmmmmmmm!

Fact 12: Peanut butter helps with weight-loss. Last thing you need to do in a survival situation is go on a deliberate diet to lose weight. But according to Richard Mattes Ph.D., R.D. and other researchers, people who ate peanut butter felt satisfied longer than other snacks. They not only felt more satisfied but lost 15-times as much weight as those that passed on food. A great snack is peanut butter on celery sticks - MMMMMmmmmm!

Fact 13: To get the tasty benefits of peanut butter it doesn't need to be cooked and that tasty peanut butter will be loyally waiting for you cause it doesn't spoil.

Fact 14: Generic brand peanut butter without the fancy name brand label is cheaper but still has the same life-saving nutrition. So buy generic peanut butter and save some $$$!

Now what are you going to buy next time you go to your favorite grocery store? Yep, get a couple bottles of that tasty peanut butter! I like the crunchy peanut butter. But remember, don't go crazy with it or you may gain a few pounds! So now you know peanut butter RULES! And you have to have some in your backpack and in your bigger static survival kits in your car, boat, trick, plane, home, cabin,... so you're ready Anytime Anywhere. Yes you can make your own peanut butter from regular peanuts if you have a high speed blender. See Vita-Mix TNT in POC Section and see peanut butter POCs in the POC Section now.

Note: I called Project Peanut Butter and was sent a 01-page note of how peanut butter is helping starving children in Malawi, Africa (southeast Africa). At the time & update of this writing (21 Feb. 2016), I'm unable to find any up-to-date referenced on Project Peanut.

Coconut Survival And More!

Now let me tell you how some survival tricks you should know about relating to coconuts. Let's start with a World Class survivor named Horace Kephart.

Kephart's Boot Waterproofing Concoctions: Kephart had several waterproofing concoctions he used on his boots and other leather ware. Here are some of his leather waterproofing concoctions.

a) Paraffin Wax & Yellow Vaseline: Melt 02 parts yellow Vaseline to 01 part paraffin wax. When in a liquid state, brush on leather.

b) Paraffin Wax & Beeswax: Melt 01 part paraffin wax to 01 part beeswax. When in a liquid state, brush on leather.

c) Paraffin Wax & Tallow: Melt 01 part paraffin wax to 01 part tallow (fat). When in a liquid state, brush on leather material for rejuvenation and protection from the elements.

d) Beeswax & Tallow: Melt 01 beeswax to 01 part tallow. When in a liquid state, brush on leather.

e) Paraffin Wax & Beeswax: Melt 01 part paraffin wax to 01 part beeswax. When in a liquid state, brush on leather.

f) Coconut Butter & Beeswax: Mix 06 parts coconut butter to 01 part beeswax. Heat to a liquid state. When in a liquid state, brush on leather.

g) Pine Tar & Cod Liver Oil: Mix and heat 02 parts pine tar and 03 parts cod liver oil. Soak the leather in the hot mixture. Rub it in. This is originally a Norwegian concoction that will make the leather waterproof and soft for months.

POW Camp Construction: Approximately 40 work camps were built by POWs between Ban Pong and Thanbyuzayat, Thailand. POWs built camps for in-coming POWs and moved 05 to 10-miles up the jungle to construct another camp. The huts in the camp were constructed using the available bamboo and giant jungle leaves (coconut palm and/or pandanus leaves). POWs demonstrated their ingenuity by building fences using bamboo. Running water was ingeniously piped in via bamboo pipes.

There were no nails to bind bamboo together so savvy POWs used strips of bark to bind the bamboo together for huts, beds, perimeter fences,... Giant jungle leaves (coconut palm and/or pandanus leaves) were used for roofing, siding, towels,... To wash and bathe themselves, POWs rubbed themselves down using cold ashes from their firepits. Rinsing off, they used jungle leaves (coconut palm and/or pandanus leaves) to dry themselves. Dug out pits were used to cook food and other dug out pits were used for latrines.

Note: Bamboo was so extremely durable, that when POWs were clearing routes for railroad tracks, it took 20 POWs all day long to clear a single clump of bamboo. At times, their Japanese captors used explosives to cut through rock, hills,...

Pacific War Canoes: Various canoes were designed and used but the long-distance war canoe was the most versatile. The war canoe had twin hulls (02 canoes side-by-side). The hulls were dug-out from tree trunks. There was a connecting platform with bamboo shelter. Twin ironwood masts and gum and matting for sails for wind propulsion. Coconut fiber rope (coir) was used in construction. Tools to construct the war canoe were axes, awls that were made from bones, shells and coral.

2nd Lt. Hiroo Onada

2nd Lt. Hiroo Onada (2003 Newsletter) of Japan did not get the word that WWII was over and he carried on the battle for approximately 30-years. Here are a few of his survival tricks including a couple that relates to coconuts.

Jungle Food: The main staple food were bananas. Banana fields were located throughout the island. Other jungle foods were citron (lemon-like fruit), **coconuts**, gaba (fruit?), mangos, nanka (fruit), papaya, pineapple, rice,...

Note: Deployed throughout Central & South America, I (author) always found wilderness food was plentiful! From bananas to mangos, it was always waiting to be picked and eaten!

Guns And Ammunition: 2nd Lt. Onoda and evaders INSURED their weapons and ammunition were well maintained for combat and hunting. Here's what they did to insure combat effectiveness:

a) Ammunition: Ammunition was placed in jars for long term storage. The ammunition was neatly stacked in the jar to get as much ammunition as possible in each jar. To insure the ammunition was airtight, **coconut oil** was poured in the jar and a lid placed on it. Jars of ammunition were cached in caves for future use. Some of the caches were so well hidden & camouflaged that the evaders often had problems recovering them.

Onoda Bamboo Fire-Starter: 2nd Lt. Onoda and evaders had another fire-starting application using bamboo, gunpowder, and tinder. Here's a step-by step using the Onoda Bamboo Fire-Starter application.

Ingredients: A section of bamboo 18 to 24-inches long, gunpowder from a bullet, and tinder (coconut fiber, or grass, or cotton fiber,...), and knife. Also have a firepit ready-to-go with tinder inside tee-pee kindling with more kindling standing-by with sustaining fuel nearby.

Step 01: Take your knife and take the section of bamboo and split it down the length so to have 02 half sections.

Step 02: Take one section and bury half of the section securely in the ground at a 45-degree. It MUST be firmly stable in the ground. Insure the edge of the bamboo is facing up.

Step 03: Take the other 1/2 section of bamboo and hold it horizontally with the inside tube of the bamboo facing up so to place & hold the gunpowder and tinder.

Step 04: Carefully place the gunpowder and tinder on top of the gunpowder in the middle of the section of bamboo.

Step 05: Holding the bamboo horizontally, take hold of it with both hands and place it on top of the bamboo section that's secured in the ground.

Step 06: Slowly start rubbing the underside of the bamboo section in your hand against the other section that's secured in the ground. INSURE the gunpowder and tinder are directly over and in-line with the other section of bamboo being rubbed against. As you slowly rub the underside of the bamboo section up & down, you'll wear a groove in the bamboo so to rub it faster and faster building-up more friction which increases the heat for ignition.

Step 07: Rub the bamboo back & forth even faster. The heat will build-up which will ignite the gunpowder which will ignite the tinder. Once ignited, carefully place the burning tinder in the nearby firepit.

Warning: Wear protective clothing, eye protection, gloves, and have natural and/or manmade fire-extinguishers standing-by.

Final Surrender / Death Statistics

Name	Date
41 soldiers	April 1946
PFC Akatsu	September 1949
Cprl Shimada	KIA 07 May 1954
PFC Kozuka	KIA 19 Oct 1972
2nd Lt. Onoda	10 March 1974

2nd Lt. Onoda stated that *"...it was my pride as an officer that sustained me during my 30 years on Lubang."* On 09 March 1974, Major Yoshimi Taniguchi read 2nd Lt. Hiroo Onoda his final military orders having him relinquish his 30-year fight on Lubang Island. On 10 March 1974, 2nd Lt. Hiroo Onoda finally surrendered. On 12 March 1974, 2nd Lt. Onoda returned to Japan to a hero's welcome. 2nd Lt. Onoda spent 19-days in Tokyo's First National Hospital. More than 200 medical tests were conducted. What doctors concluded was that 2nd Lt. Onoda's mental and physical health was superior to his peers who lived in city environments.

This concludes 2nd Lt. Onoda's and his comrades survival applications, techniques, and tricks. I know you learned some real wilderness survival from a Japanese legend and here comes some more so you're ready Anytime Anywhere!

Coconut Research & Development (R & D) Notes!

a) Coconut Shell & Fiber: I found coconut shell fiber to ignite and burn very readily and with good ignition. The shell holds a good burning ember. I took sections of the coconut shell, added 07 fish oil capsules and it easily ignited. It also ignited without any additional oil. Also as times goes on with the coconut shell open and drying, the coconut meat separates from the coconut shell (03-days).

b) Coconut Milk: Provided about 02 fluid ounces (03 good swallows) of tasty coconut milk.

c) Coconut Meat: Coconut meat was extremely tasty. Small sections of coconut meat easily ignited and displayed fireworks! Why? The coconut meat contains coconut oil.

d) Flotation: Coconut shell (de-husked) floats with 3/4 of it submerged. Would take at least 40-50 to support a non or weak swimmer. I submerged a de-husked coconut in water. On day 14, its still floating. See Item 185 - Coconut Fireworks.

Coconut Survival Use: The coconut palm (also called coco, coco palm, coconut tree) tree is found in tropical regions. An adult coconut tree clocks-in at 18-inches in diameter with a height of 100-feet.

At the summit (top) of the coconut tree grows approximately 20 pinnate leaves (10-15 feet) generally curved downward. Here, several clusters of coconuts in different levels of maturity grow in clusters of 10-20 nuts. The mature coconut is approximately 12-inches long with a thick fibrous husk that protects a hard inner shell we know as the coconut. One single coconut tree can produce 50+ coconuts per year! Coconuts have several survival uses and here are 2nd. Lt. Onoda's survival tricks and a few more you have to know:

a) **Food:** The white flesh of the coconut provides nutrients as well as healthy oil. The center stem of a young palm is edible and succulent. Palm cabbage is also a food source and considered a delicacy. Adult coconut trees are cut down to get to the palm cabbage.

b) **Oil:** Oil is taken from the white flesh of coconut called copra. The coconut oil was used to oil weapons. It can also be used for cooking, fuel for fire, and as a cosmetic for skin. The white, oily meat is dried to produce the commercially valuable copra which provides oil to produce candles, cosmetics, soap,... See *Coconut Fireworks*.

c) **Coconut Milk:** The white sweet coconut milk can be consumed without filtering or purifying. Also used for cooking.

d) Coconut Tree Sap: The sap or *"toddy"* is gathered and consumed as a favorite drink. It is also fermented and distilled to produce a favorite alcoholic drink called palm wine or arrack.

e) Bed Matting: The outer fibers of the coconut can be gathered for bed matting.

f) Leaves: The dried leaves are used to weave baskets, mats, screens,... The leaves are also used for thatching (for building shelters and roofing). Believe it or not, modern day houses are thatched instead of using conventional roofing because its proven its worth against the elements.

g) Flotation: Coconuts with the protecting husk float. Secure a bunch together (20+) and they'll temporarily support a survivor while resting or doing the dog paddle in deep water.

h) Bait: The flesh white coconut can be used for bait in conjunction with properly built & located traps and snares designed for a particular small or big game.

i) Coconut Palm Root: The roots possess a narcotic. The roots are chewed to induce an intoxication.

j) Rope: The fibers from the outer husk (also called coir) are weaved to make rope. And believe me, it will make a strong rope. I and others made a rope from grass and its practically unbreakable. Yes, it takes time weaving it, but it's a surprisingly STRONG rope.

k) Coconut Lees: 2nd Lt. was always aware of several species of nagging, biting, stinging ants. To keep the ants away, he placed small piles of coconut lees (sediment of coconut milk after it was heated) several meters away from his shelter. The ants went for the sweet coconut lees instead of bothering him.

l) Coconut Shell: The coconut shell can be used for various containers and formed into different tools. Remember *"Necessity is the mother of invention."*

1st WARNING: The last place to stand, rest, sleep,... is under a coconut palm tree. A full grown coconut weighs-in at 7+- pounds and with a 100-foot fall, that 07-pound coconut could reach a velocity that could kill you dead if it hits you in the right place. At minimum it'll put a hurtn' on you so bad that you'll be cussing every coconut tree for a 100-miles around! Can you imagine laying there face-up, minding your own business, eyes closed, taking in the beauty of Mother Nature and P O W - you get BASHED by a 07-pound coconut square in the face!

2nd WARNING: While I'm at it, soldiers pulling security under tall trees have been KILLED DEAD from falling dead tree limbs and falling trees. So before you settle down at night (02-hours before dusk), look up and inspect the tree for dead limbs and inspect the surround tress for sturdiness.

In 1989 while at Ft. Davis, Panama, one day I was running some extra miles on a semi-lone road to Dock 45. Wearing my walkman, I heard a crash directly behind me. Tearing off my headset, I looked back to find a bunch of heavy limbs still swaying on the pavement from the crash. Those heavy limbs missed me by a couple seconds. I remember telling myself "It could have killed me...!" If I wasn't killed immediately, I probably would have died from my wounds cause the road is real quiet on weekends. I would have layed there many minutes to several hours before help arrived. So again, LOOK-UP and check the tree above you for dead limbs and check tree sturdiness before you set camp - they could fall on you causing serious injuries or death.

Coconut Fire-Starting R & D!

Now let me cover some more advanced fire-starting applications you have to know cause they could save your life Anytime Anywhere! Let's start with Coconut Fireworks!

Coconut Fireworks: Now here's a different fire-starting application using coconuts. You learned from 2nd Lt. Onoda's 30-year evasion that he used coconut fiber as tinder.

But nowhere in my research did I find 01 single word about those evaders using the sweet tasting coconut meat itself or the coconut shell for fire-starting. Here's my own Research & Development (R&D).

Coconut Shell: The coconut shell is a great fuel. It doesn't take much to ignite the hard dry shell. Once lit, it has a little fireworks to it and seems to shootout gases. This is probably from coconut oil within the shell. One thing about the coconut shell, once the fire is extinguished, the shell smolders for a surprisingly long time. Its red glow is very bright and easily seen even during daylight hours. The long smoldering coconut shell can be used to ignite tinder.

Coconut Meat: The delicious sweet coconut meat is a very good fuel! Why? Because of the coconut oil within the white meat. I fired-up a piece of white coconut meat the size of my thumb. The meat wasn't dry and still damp from the coconut milk. Even though I had no real trouble igniting the wet coconut meat with a match, no doubt it would fire-up even quicker if it was bone dry. Once ignited, it displayed the best and most beautiful fireworks I have ever seen.

With its loud cracking and popping sounds, it continuously spit out dark sky-blue pellets of fire. It also shot out specks of fire that exploded inches away from the coconut meat leaving circles of smoke. This small piece of coconut meat the size of my thumb burnt for 05 minutes and 30 seconds.

One day I'll take a whole coconut (white meat and shell) and fire it up! I know it will burn real good (Advanced Fire-Starting Video Part V??). Now you know coconuts are not only a good food source, they're also great fuel source for a life-saving fires! Now here's another advanced fire-starting application you never heard of - only from IRISAP!

Coconut Fire-Starting Applications (02)!

Coconut Fire-Starting #01: You read about my coconut R&D on pages 30 and 40. I'm really surprised 2nd Lt. Hiroo Onoda during his 30-years of evasion and survival didn't use coconuts as a fuel source for fires. As you'll read, all you need is a coconut! No kindling, no sustaining fuel - just coconuts!

Ingredients: A coconut, coconut fiber, flint for sparks, cotton t-shirt, and knife.

Step 01: Take your coconut and gather the tinder around the shell and set it aside for later. If there's not enough, grab a 1/2-handful of dry grass tinder.

Step 02: Take your coconut. You'll notice on one end is a face having 03 holes which represent 02 eyes and a mouth. Take your knife and drill a hole in one of the eyes or the mouth and drain the coconut milk. Once it's drained, break the coconut in half.

Step 03: You can separate the white meat from the shell using a knife or you can let both halves dry for about 10-14 days. If drying, the white meat will automatically separate itself from the coconut shell. Once dry, you may have to pry it here and there but coconut meat separates intact from the coconut shell.

Step 04: Take your knife and cut thin slices out of the coconut meat from 01 to 06 inches long. To make slicing easier, you can break the halves into quarters. The sliced coconut meat burns very well plus it will burn for a long time (keep reading). You should end up with a pile of thin coconut slices.

Step 05: Take your t-shirt and secure it on your lap. Take your knife and scrape back & forth 50-times across the t-shirt. Collect the fine fiber off your knife, pants, hands, arms,... using the blade of your knife and secure it to the side. Continue scraping again for another 50 and collect the fine cotton fiber. Continue till you have a ball of it the size of a ping pong. Yes, you can use the cotton ball from one of the several survival kits I sent you.

Step 06: Take a coconut shell half and go to the face and drill holes in the other 02 holes. Then you'll have 03 drilled holes in the face. Drill the holes so they're 1/2-inch wide.   The drilled holes will provide additional oxygen to the fire.

Step 07: Take your cotton ball and fluff it up. From the inside of the coconut shell place a small portion of the cotton ball through one of the drilled holes. It will be lit from outside the shell using sparks.

Step 08: Place your coconut tinder and or grass tinder inside the coconut shell and place it on top of the fluffed-up cotton ball.

Step 09: Place about 09 slices of coconut slices on top of the tinder. Insure all slices are separated and not stacked.

Step 10: The coconut shell acts as a safe container for the fire. You can initially carry it to a designated area or carve a small depression in the ground to secure it.

Step 11: To light the fire, go to the bottom of the coconut shell where cotton is sticking out of one of the 03 drilled holes. Using your expended lighter, throw some sparks at it. This will lite the cotton which will burn thru the drilled hole igniting the cotton ball. The cotton ball will ignite the tinder. The flaming tinder will ignite the 09 slices of coconut meat. Once the slices of coconut meat are ignited, they burn very well. The burn is hot, bright, with flames about 07-inches high and complimented with tiny fireworks with cracklings and pops.

1st Note: When igniting the cotton tinder, it is very vulnerable to any wind. So when igniting it, protect it from the wind even a slight breeze. YES, if you want you can use a match or lighter!

After 03-minutes or when needed, add 03 more slices of coconut meat to sustain the fire. With all the slices from just one coconut, if you place 03 slices in the coconut shell every 03-minutes, the fire should burn up to 90-minutes! And don't forget, the coconut shell burns too!

2nd Note: If there's an Advanced Fire-Starting Video Part V, you'll definitely see this in the video.

3rd Note: Went outside (301233C January 2003) to retrieve the half coconut shell. Couldn't find it anywhere, with a fenced-in yard some critter jumped over or went under the fence with it. Why would any critter want an empty 1/2 coconut shell and with burned coconut slices in it? Probably a *"nekko!"* (Japanese for cat - 2nd Lt. Onoda - get it). Anyway want another and easier fire-starting application using a coconut? OK, let's get started.

4th Note: Listen if you don't want to light the cotton tinder as prescribed above, read the next application for easier ignition.

Coconut Fire-Starting #02: This next similar application is easier to fire-up and burn than the 1st one.

Ingredients: A coconut, flint for sparks, cotton t-shirt, and knife.

Step 01: Take your coconut. You'll notice on one end is a face having 03 holes which represent 02 eyes and a mouth. Take your knife and drill a hole in one of the eyes or the mouth and drain the coconut milk. Once it's drained, break the coconut in half.

Step 02: Separate the white meat from the shell by DRYING ONLY - we want both coconut meat halves intact for right now. Let both halves dry for about 10-14 days. The white meat will automatically separate itself from the coconut shell. Once dry, you may have to pry it here and there but coconut meat separates intact from the coconut shell.

Step 03: Using ONLY one of the halves, take your knife and cut thin slices out of the coconut meat from 01 to 06 inches long. To make slicing easier, you can break the half into two parts. The sliced coconut meat burns very well plus it will burn for a long time (keep reading). You should end up with a pile of thin coconut slices.

Step 04: Take your t-shirt and secure it on your lap. Take your knife and scrape back & forth 50-times across the t-shirt. Collect the fine fiber off your knife, pants, hands, arms,... using the blade of your knife and secure it to the side. Continue scraping again for another 50 and collect the fine cotton fiber. Continue till you have a ball of it the size of a ping pong. Yes, you can use the cotton ball from one of the several survival kits I sent you.

Step 05: Take a coconut meat half and go to the face and drill holes in the other 02 holes. Then you'll have 03 drilled holes in the face. However, for this fire-starting application, drill 03 more holes for adequate air. All fires need heat, fuel, and oxygen and this application requires plenty of oxygen. The extra drilled holes will provide additional oxygen to the fire.

Step 06: Take your cotton ball and fluff it up. Take several coconut slices and place them next to your side within fast grasp. Ignite the fluffed-up cotton ball with sparks (expended flint lighter) and drop it in the coconut meat half. IMMEDIATELY take one of the coconut slices to the burning cotton ball and ignite it. It will sweat and ignite in about 01 or 02 seconds max. Once it's burning place it in the coconut meat half and add 08 more coconut slices.

Step 07: Once all 08 coconut slices are burning, carefully place 12 more coconut slices for a sure a good fire build-up.

Do not stack them - stagger and separate them. Once the 12 slices of coconut meat are ignited, they'll burn real good. The burn is hot, bright, with flames about 07-inches high and complimented with tiny fireworks with cracklings and pops. This will build-up the heat high enough so that the coconut half will start burning. Once the coconut meat half starts burning, it will burn for approximately 34-minutes with a hot flame that's bright reaching 07 or so inches high. The coconut burned in a moderate wind. With a calm or no wind, burn time could reach 40 to 45 minutes.

Step 08: The coconut meat half acts as a safe container for the fire. You can initially carry it to a designated area or carve a small depression in the ground to secure it. And remember, you still have all those other slices of coconut meat for fuel and vittles. As in the 1st fire-starting application, piece-mealing slices of coconut will have the fire burning for 90-minutes or more!

Note: YES, if you want you can use a match or lighter!

One main difference between this fire-starting application and the coconut shell half is the coconut meat half itself will eventually IGNITE (within a minute) for a good fire without feeding the fire every 03-minutes or so.

So next time you go out camping, take a few coconuts with you! And besides, coconuts satisfy all *8 Elements of Survival* (Fire, Water, Shelter, First-Aid, Signal, Food, Weapons, and Navigation).

Black Gold African Tea: Many years, natives living near an African swamp, skimmed the black liquid from the surface of the swamp water. The black liquid was fuel to light their huts. They stated to their white observers that the black liquid was given to them by the Sun God. The black liquid was actually oil. The natives gathered the oil in coconut shells, gourds,... Pouring the oil in small containers and using liana (woody vine) for wicks, the oil provided FREE FUEL to light their homes.

Coconut Cooking Pot: You already read how I used a coconut shell, coconut fiber, cotton t-shirt, coconut meat, and some sparks,... to start a life-saving fire in the 2003 Newsletter. You've seen many a fake survivors drinking and eating from coconut shells on TV and the movies. But what about a cooking pot using a coconut shell? Can it be done? Well let me show you how it's done boiling 03 large eggs and frying 03 large eggs in the Coconut Cooking Pot. Let's start with the necessary Ingredients.

Boiling Eggs!

Ingredients: Coconuts (02), saw blade, sharp knife (utility knife), butter knife, spoon, tee-pee firepit, 06 fresh eggs, and water.

Step 01: Construct a tee-pee kindling firepit with plenty of grass tinder. Ignite and keep adding kindling as needed for a good bed of coals.

Meanwhile, while the kindling is burning and the hot coals are being built-up...

Step 02: Go to the 03 holes in the face (02 eyes and mouth) of the coconut and pierce the eye closest to the top of the coconut. More times than not this is always the easiest hole to penetrate. Once an aperture is made, drain the coconut milk and drink or save for future use.

Step 03: As I stated in Coconut R&D in the 2003 Newsletter, as the coconut ages, it will automatically start splitting around the middle circumference of the coconut shell. If this is the case use the splitting line as a guide and saw the coconut shell completely around the circumference of the coconut without sawing it in half. You're just scarring the coconut. Stand up and drop the coconut at waist level once or twice to a hard surface and it should open in two equal halves - more or less. More times than not it will break in 02 equally formed halves.

However, if you're in a hurry, just drop the coconut at waist level on a hard surface and it should break in two halves and not necessarily equal halves.

Step 04: Take your sharp knife and carefully make 10 evenly spaced lengthwise cuts from the bottom center to the outer rim. Make a few more horizontal cuts intersecting the vertical cuts in both coconut halves.

Note: If unable to make intersecting cuts, just cut as you go and excavate each piece of coconut meat for both halves.

Step 05: Take your butter knife and carefully excavate the coconut meat without breaking the coconut halves. After excavating all the coconut meat, refrigerate it for future food and/or you can use it as fuel. Both coconut shell halves should be about 1/8th of an inch wide. Repeat all Steps with the 2nd coconut.

IMPORTANT NOTE: Only 01 of the 02 halves can be used as a Coconut Cooking Pot. Why? Because the half with the face (03 holes) is soft and will eventually leak anyway. That's why we need two coconuts to get 02 Coconut Cooking Pots.

Note: If you keep the coconut meat at room temperature, it will mold within 48-hours.

Step 06: Add 06-fluid ounces of water to the coconut bowl till it's about half-way filled. Place 03 large eggs in the bowl. Add more water if necessary.

Step 07: Carefully place the Coconut Cooking Pot and its contents in the fire and eventually in the center of the firepit within the bed of red hot coals so it's surrounded by intense heat for faster boiling.

Step 08: The water will heat to a high temperature but not to a rolling boil. The water will heat to a stirring, steaming motion with small bubbles. There will be some evaporation.

Step 09: I boiled 03 large eggs in 25-minutes. The eggs were cooked like I like them, the egg white cooked - not runny and the yolks soft. The Coconut Cooking Pot was charred, damaged and started leaking at 25-minutes. I do not recommend using it again as a cooking pot. It can still be used as a container. (R&D conducted on 12 July 2003)

Scrambling Eggs!

Step 10: The other Coconut Cooking Pot, I placed upside down in the fire for about 30-seconds to kill any germs, bacteria,...

Step 11: I cooked some fresh scrambled eggs in this 2nd half. I poured 03 large eggs (stirred) in the coconut shell and placed it in the fire. Stirring occasionally, at 10-minutes, I could hear the eggs frying against the inside walls of the Coconut Cooking Pot. The scrambled eggs were cooked in only 13-minutes.

After cooking, the coconut shell was charred, damaged, and prone to leaking. I do not recommend using it as a cooking pot again. At 02 to 06-minutes after the Coconut Cooking Pot was removed from the fire, it was crackling due to cooling down, or water causing expansion..

1st Note: Now you know how to cook using Coconut Cooking Pots over an open fire. The drawback is that they can only be used one time. Keep reading to see how to use the Coconut Cooking Pot multiple times.

2nd Note: With the other 02 coconut shells with the faces (03 holes), use them as containers for non-fluid items.

Scrambling Eggs In Water!

Here's a technique using the Coconut Cooking Pot to cook meals without damaging it so you can use it again and again.

Step 12: If you already have a metal pot, you can cook scrambled eggs and many other meals in water. Get some water to boil in a 06-inch deep pot (minimum).

Step 13: Take the Coconut Cooking Pot and carefully dip it in the boiling water 02 or 03 times to kill any germs, bacteria,...

Step 14: Stir 03 fresh eggs and pour them into the Coconut Cooking Pot AWAY from the boiling water.

Step 15: Secure the Coconut Cooking Pot with its contents (03 stirred eggs) and carefully place it in the boiling water. Do not drop it in for it will capsize.

Step 16: Do not disturb or stir the eggs for you may cause the Coconut Cooking Pot to capsize. Add water to the metal pot if necessary for the Coconut Cooking Pot MUST CONTINUOUSLY FLOAT to maintain its buoyancy and especially balance to avoid capsizing. It will take approximately 01-hour 26-minutes for the 03 fresh eggs to cook to a scrambled egg consistency. Compare the time of cooking scrambled eggs over an open fire (13-minutes) over an open fire, the Coconut Cooking Pot is not only charred but also damaged and good for a one time use.

1st Note: You can use this slow cooking technique to cook many small meals, make stews, make soups, make teas, make coffee, make cocoa,... and the best part about using this technique versus using the Coconut Cooking Pot over an open fire is that it's NOT damaged by intense heat and can be used over and over again.

2nd Note: Depending on the size of your metal cooking pot, you can use this same technique to prepare several meals simultaneously using several Coconut Cooking Pots.

Important Note: DO NOT pour the 03 fresh eggs in the Coconut Cooking Pot while it's floating in the boiling water. The unbalanced load will capsize the Coconut Cooking Pot pouring the stirred eggs in the water.

Now you know how to cook using tsama melons, cantaloupes, and coconut shells as cooking pots. YES, there are many fruits, vegetables, animal skulls (stoves),... you can use as cooking pots as I stated on the previous page.

Coconut Candle: Here's one of the longest burning oils and it's a delicious oil you can eat - coconut oil. In Advanced Fire-Starting Videos Parts III and IV, you saw plenty of examples using various oils and fats to make super cheap candles, light reflectors, stoves, torches,... I gave you plenty of time hacks for those various oils and fats to show you their long burn time. And coconut oil is another long burning oil. Just watch those Survival Videos to use coconut oil for candles, light reflectors, stoves, torches,...

Approximately 02-fluid ounces of coconut oil burns approximately 04-hours and 49-minutes. At room temperature coconut oil has milky white blotches with some clear oil. When refrigerated, it turns into a solid white mass resembling paraffin wax. A 14-ounce jar of coconut oil costs about $05.43 at local health food stores.

When ignited, the coconut oil burns a bright 01-inch to 02-inch flame with some black smoke. At 02-hrs 22-mins, I swapped to the other tail-end of the 06-inch cotton t-shirt wick for a renewed flame. At 04-hrs 03-mins and 04-hrs 30-mins, I carefully pulled out the cotton t-shirt wick to renew the flame. I also tilted the aluminum can (soda can) to burn all remaining coconut oil. Total burn time for 02-fluid ounces of coconut oil - 04-hours 49-minutes.

1st Note: Flame is fragile and should be used indoors. Straighten-out paperclip and pull out wick to renew flame. Capillary action sucks-up all the coconut oil to the wick to burn. Wick burned-out with remaining wick still saturated. Approximately 10 drops of coconut oil remaining.

2nd Note: Coconut oil (warm) is delicious. I've cooked with it and ate it with bread. And here's the best part, it's a Medium Chain Triglyceride (MCT) meaning it will help you lose weight if you're overweight.

Coconut Ratio Formula!

I told you how long 02-fluid ounces will burn. But how long can a bottle of 14 fluid ounces of coconut oil burn? Here's a Ratio Formula we'll use. Use Ratio Formula for just about anything:

Step 01:

02 fluid oz = 289 minutes
---------- ----------
14 fluid oz = ??? minutes

Step 02:

289 X 14 = 4,046

Step 03:

4046 ÷ 02 = 2,023

Step 04:

2,023 total minutes ÷ 60 = 33.71666 or approximately 33+ hours. So 14 fluid ounces of coconut oil will burn approximately 33 hours (01 wick)! And read about the long burn time of canola oil on page 53. While we're on the subject of coconuts, let's carry-on with some more Coconut R&D.

More Coconut R & D: I conducted some more coconut research & development I thought you should know about.

a) Rotting Coconut: If a coconut is left whole with its milk intact, the coconut will begin rotting after approximately 06-weeks. A week or so later, the coconut will show a crack from the inside along its equator but the shell may still be intact. The coconut milk is brownish yellow and is NOT consumable. The entire coconut meat turns a golden brown color, is mushy soft with a mild odor and is NOT edible.

If the soft coconut is allowed to dry, it is still ignitable? According to my own R&D – it's very ignitable. It's still soft compared to fresh coconut meat but very ignitable. Because it was mushy, it may gather a greenish mold after a few days to a week. The mold acts as a fire retardant. Just scrape away the mold and the mushy coconut meat should ignite with GREAT FIREWORKS complimented with popping, crackling, and spitting fire!

Warning: The greenish mold is not ignitable. The survivor may be allergic to the mold causing mild to serious health problems.

b) Coconut Meat: After draining a coconut, 10-weeks later, the coconut meat is discolored and is almost completely overtaken and *"eaten"* by a black mold. The meat partially detaches itself from the shell. The meat is still very ignitable. Just cut white pieces not eaten by the black mold. When cutting away the coconut meat, you can still see the coconut oil at the surface. It burns great and complimented with fireworks of crackling, popping, spitting fire,...

Warning: The fluffy black mold is not ignitable. The survivor may be allergic to the mold causing mild to serious health problems.

c) Coconut Shell: 10-weeks after draining the coconut milk, the shell remains almost indestructible, waterproof, and ignitable.

d) Fresh Coconut: The moral to all this Coconut R&D - use FRESH coconuts if possible. On your next outdoor adventure, purchase FRESH coconuts (less than $1 each) cause they satisfy all *8 Elements of Survival* (Fire, Water, Shelter, First-Aid, Signal, Food, Weapons, and Navigation). And they'll last throughout your outdoor adventure as long as you don't stay out there several weeks!

Asian Coconut Fire-Starting: Asian Coconuts, also called Young Coconuts are actually coconuts you've bought in the store but are harvested much earlier (keep reading). The regular *"coconuts"* you've been purchasing in the store are actually called "old coconuts"! That's exactly what an Asian lady told me when I was trying to figure out the difference between Asian Coconuts and regular coconuts. Anyway, here's a fire-starting application using Asian Coconuts (Young Coconuts). OK, let's get started with Ingredients.

Ingredients: Asian coconut - it's white cause the outer skin has been cut away - you're actually looking at the white husk and it may be pointed at one end. Looks soft but it's tough. You'll also need a butcher knife, spoon, garden shears (I have a set in my bigger survival kit), 01 match, firepit with tinder (not really necessary), wood kindling, and sustaining fuel.

Step 01: Carefully carve away the outer white husk. Continue to carve till you notice at one end of the coconut is very soft and pliable. This is the end you'll make an aperture to retrieve the coconut milk.

Step 02: Carefully carve a small hole in this soft part of the coconut and drain the coconut milk into a clean container. You'll get an amazing 11-ounces! Yes, you can drink it - I did!

Note: Old coconuts (more mature) have about 07-ounces of coconut milk versus 11-ounces of 'young coconuts.'

Step 03: Once you drained the coconut milk, drink it or store it in a sealed container and put in a cool place (life-span is short). Keep carving away the white husk till you meet hard resistance of the shell.

Step 04: Insert your garden shears into the small aperture and begin cutting away into the shell around the circumference of the coconut.

Step 05: Once the coconut shell is cut in half, you'll notice the inside of both halves is made-up of a thin white layer of coconut meat that's about 1/8th of an inch wide or less. The coconut meat is very tender like oysters and it's very delicious. I ate some but had to stop myself to use it as fuel.

Step 06: Cut away the tender thin coconut meat. You can eat it, or let it dry out for a long-term food source (MUST refrigerate) and as a fuel source - kindling. To cut away the coconut meat from the bottom center of both halves, you'll need a spoon to cut and scoop it out. If you want, use the spoon to carve out all the very tender coconut meat.

Step 07: The thin coconut meat may take a week to dry but is still moist-looking and pliable due to the coconut oil (fuel) within it. After the thin coconut meat is 'dry,' it's ready as quick-burning kindling. I DO NOT recommend that you eat it - taste terrible after it's been dried-out for a week.

Step 08: The slices of young coconut are great kindling. Once a match is put to them, they'll fire-up complimented by fireworks, crackling, and popping.

1st Note: The tender thin coconut meat must be dried-out for it to fire-up. It won't ignite just out of the shell because it's wet with coconut milk.

2nd Note: The outer white husk is kinda tough. It's non-flammable when moist or dried-out, I couldn't get it to burn, but it's buoyant. However, when fresh if you chew and suck on it, you can draw-out some sweet coconut juice - it's DELICIOUS! An Asian lady told me you can eat the outer husk! She said to cut it in slices and eat them raw or cook them. I'd like to run into her again and get more cooking tips on Asian Coconuts.

I'd really like to see her eat the husk. Anyway, the coconut shell can also be used to satisfy the *8 Elements of Survival* (Fire, Water, Shelter, First-Aid, Signal, Food, Weapons, and Navigation).

3rd Note: Coconut husk in non-flammable but buoyant. I've soaked pieces of it for 20-hours and it still floats but tends to sink. As you already know from the 2003 Newsletter Coconut R&D, whole 'old coconuts' intact are very buoyant and stay buoyant for long periods of time.

4th Note: What about coconut husk wicks you ask? No way, as I've stated the husk is non-flammable. I've tried to light coconut husk wicks but they burn out real quick. But the brown coconut fiber from "old coconuts" make great emergency wicks! Just wad it making a 02-inch wick and secure it to the wick holder (aluminum triangle wick holder - see Advanced Fire-Starting Video Part III). The brown coconut fiber wick burned for a surprising 16-hours and that's because it burned all but a few drops of the 02-fluid ounces of canola oil. It would have burned more if I added more fuel (canola oil).

Doing a ratio problem, 02 fluid ounces of canola oil = 16-hours of burn time so a 24-ounce bottle of canola oil has an approximate burn time of 192-hours or 08 days & nights (24-hours a day). And the bottle of canola oil cost only $1.15.

So you got plenty of SAFE fuel (non-explosive) for your next outdoor adventure! The longer it burned, the better the flame (wide flame). The wick kinda spread out (wide flame) a bit but still produced a single bright flame.

The long burn time of coconut fiber surprised even me and it burned very clean - NO SMOKE! I went shopping for some canola oil. At a local Shop N Save grocery store, I found a 128-fluid ounce bottle (01 gallon) of Shop N Save Canola Oil for only $4.19. Doing a ratio problem, that 128-fluid ounce bottle of canola oil will burn approximately 1,024-hours or 42 days!

YES, you can find even cheaper or FREE fuel like the fat butchers throw away, cooking fats and oils in your own kitchen. And what about all that discarded oil from fast food restaurants (Mc Donalds, Hardees, Burger King, Dairy Queen, KFC, Popeye's, Church's Chicken, restaurants,...)?

Again, I was using canola oil as fuel and there are a dozen more oils, fats,... you can use as fuel.   I'm sure there are other "fibrous-type" wicks you can use in your neck of the woods. I still like using a piece of cotton t-shirt for emergency wicks cause they're readily available (odds are you're wearing cotton underwear right now) and have a long burn time. See Advanced Fire-Starting Videos Parts III & IV for making FREE candles, heaters, light reflectors, stoves,... for your next outdoor adventure.

5th Note: My BEST recommendation is to use "old coconuts" on your outdoor adventures cause they have PLENTY of fuel, and satisfy all 8 Elements of Survival (fire, water, shelter, first-aid, signal, food, weapons, and navigation). SEE the 2003 Newsletter for more Coconut Fire-Starting and R&D! See Fire-Starting & Fires! in the A-Z Index now.

Now that you've had plenty of fire-starting throughout this Newsletter, let's see how to fight killer cold temperatures like Indians, mountain men and a lone magician. WAIT - found some lost R&D!

Lost Coconut R & D!
Here's some lost R&D I misplaced. Thought you'd like to have it cause it's real workable survival so you're ready Anytime Anywhere.

Coconut Kindling: I just found some lost Coconut R & D. Approximately 02 months ago back about 19 May 2003, I took a coconut half and took it apart. I broke up the shell and placed it in a zip lock bag. I took the coconut meat and cut it into many thin slices and placed them in the ziplock bag too. With the ziplock bag being airtight, 02-months later, there was absolutely no evidence of mold on any of the coconut meat.

As I stated before, if you leave fresh coconut meat out in the open air (indoors or outdoors), it will begin to harbor mold in about 48-hours.

And mold acts as a fire retardant, plus it ain't healthy to a lot of allergic folks. Anyway, the thin sliced-up coconut meat appeared to be dried out yet if you break it or pierce it with a knife, paperclip, pushpin,... you'll still find it's loaded with oozing coconut oil (ignitable fuel). I took one thin slice of coconut meat (about the length of my small finger) and lit it with a single match.

In just a second or two it took off as expected and was complimented with pops, crackling, and spitting 4th of July fireworks of different colors (better seen at night). That small thin slice of coconut meat burned for 01-minute and 15-seconds (75-seconds). The dried sliced coconut meat is great kindling. YES, it was still edible and tasty too after 02-months in the ziplock bag! Yes, you can use it for critter bait, first-aid (skin),...

As I stated before, consider carrying fresh coconuts on all your outdoor adventures cause they satisfy all *08 Elements of Survival* (Fire, Water, Shelter, First-Aid, Signal, Food, Weapons, and Navigation.) YES, I talked to one of them produce guys at the grocery store - coconuts ARE AVAILABLE all the time - throughout the year, at your local grocery store! PLEASE re-read all Coconut R&D, Coconut Fire-Starting, and general Coconut Survival Data throughout the 2003 Newsletter, 2004 Newsletter, and other Newsletter s (see A-Z Index).

Lyon's Cocoon Hammock: Here's an invention of Mr. Lyons and he got the idea from a caterpillar inside its cocoon. Years ago, Mr. Lyons invented the Lyon's Cocoon Hammock.

It was a hammock and sleeping bag together instead of a plain ol' sleeping bag layed out on top of a hammock like we've all used before. And to smartly compliment the Lyon's Cocoon Hammock, a mosquito net, insulation and a waterproof sleeve were also part of the ingenious Lyon's Cocoon Hammock. Sounds like the Lyon's Cocoon Hammock is ready Anytime Anywhere!

WARNING: Before setting-up any campsite, look above for the status of trees and vegetation above. Falling deadfall will kill you dead or at best send you to the local ER. Never never rest or sleep under palm trees where coconuts are growing. It's estimated that **150 people per year are KILLED BY FALLING COCONUTS!** That's 10-times more people killed by them ornery sharks!

Fertig Chicken Meal: As the roasting red pigs (lechon) were rotated over the hot bed of coals, melting pig grease dripped onto the coals creating more burning fuel to roast the pigs. But another part of the dinner were the chickens. Over smaller fires, chickens were split open and stuffed with camotes. The roasted chickens were rotated till the meat and camotes were thoroughly roasted. For you military types, odds are you'll run into plenty of chickens before you run into pigs (wild or tame). And don't forget the several techniques on Hypnotizing Chickens for silent humane kills - see the A-Z Index.

1st Note: Fertig and his comrades were lucky enough to partake in several foods provided by the jungle and the friendly villagers. Other foods included: avocados, bananas, casava roots, coconut meat, coconut milk, crayfish, fern tips, fish, fresh-water shrimp, jackfruit, large roasted seeds, locusts, monkeys, muscavado sugar, pamelos, pineapples, rats, rough-cracked corn, white rice, wild boars, wild pigeon,...

2nd Note: Freshwater shrimp (white fish) found in rivers were caught by hand. It was best cooked with coarse-salt and sweet-potato leaves.

In the 1st Note above, I told you Fertig's men captured and ate wild boar. Before I forget, let me tell you about the Georgia Wild Boar Stunner.

Fertic Polished Wood: Here's a technique to polish wood which might come in handy. Who knows - you just never know. In this case, this technique was used to polish the wooden floors of a prominent villager. Women secured coconut husks to their feet. With coconut husks secured to their feet, the women skated over the floor. Doing this daily chore, the floor shined, thus giving the dwelling an air of royalty.

Fertig Battery Recharger: Telephone batteries could not be replaced. Amazingly, it was discovered how to recharge the batteries. The telephone batteries were submerged in tuba (coconut beer) overnight.

Amazingly, the battery recharged. This Fertig Battery Recharger was so effective it was used by all the resistance forces throughout the Philippines.

Laydon's Battery Recharger R & D: I thought the Fertig Battery Recharger was worthy of some R&D (Research & Development) so here it is (092000C February 2007).

I took 03 Panasonic AA batteries and ran them in a small RadioShack radio. Once the batteries were run down to nothing, I kept the radio on for another 12 hours. The 03 AA batteries were dead dead - no life to them whatsoever.

I then took a cold bottle of beer - a 12-fluid ounce of Samuel Adams Cherry Wheat beer and took a good swallow from it (MMmmmmmmm) to adjust for the volume for replacement of the 03 batteries. I dropped the 03 dead batteries in the bottle of beer and they hit the bottom of the glass bottle. Immediately beer foam came pouring out of the top of the bottle. Enough foam that I had a little cleaning up to do.

Foam covered the top of the bottle and I replaced the bottle cap (non twist off). To insure I got a half way decent seal on the bottle I placed a small section of Glad Press'n Seal over the bottle cap and top neck of the glass bottle. I placed the beer bottle in a glass bowl in case it overflowed and placed everything in the fridge. The 03 *"dead"* batteries remained in the bottle for approximately 16-hours.

I removed the 03 *"dead"* AA batteries from the bottle of beer. Drying them off, I then placed the batteries in my small RadioShack radio and turned it on. The radio responded to a LOUD volume. After finding a Country Western channel, I noticed the 03 batteries quickly losing their power. However, even at a low volume, the 03 rejuvenated batteries kept the radio playing for 30 minutes! Not bad from dead dead dead batteries to rejuvenated batteries! Wait!

After 30-minutes of running the radio, the volume and reception became weak so I turned off the radio to see if the 03 batteries could recover like most batteries do. After 60-minutes of rest, I turned on the radio and sure enough, the 03 batteries re-rejuvenated themselves. I continued to do this and the batteries recovered again and again. Timing these 03 *"dead"* batteries, I had a total running time (weak) of 01-hour 23-minutes. Not bad uh!

That may not seem like a long time but in emergency situations, I think the Fertig Battery Recharger survival trick may give your radio (receiving radio signals) or Walkie-Talkie (transmit emergency message(s) just enough power to get you out of trouble and save your life and those comrades under your command Anytime Anywhere!

1st Note: Holding the radio near the body aids in reception. And knowing the directional source of the signal may help out too.

2nd Note: I'm not sure if the yeast in beer aids to rejuvenate batteries or what. I also don't know about how this same application will apply to all sorts of other batteries. It's beyond my own R&D (time & money).

Tapping Battery Recharger: If Tapping Battery Recharger: I thought I'd add this recharging trick in here. Even though I haven't conducted any R&D on it to prove or disprove it - I thought it be worthy of your attention. An insurance inspector was out here inspecting the roof (March 2008). His flashlight was going dim so to recharge the batteries real quick, he removed the batteries and tapped the negative ends of each battery against each other. Sure enough, the light beam was stronger than before! Do your own R&D and let me know what happened.

Fertig Soap: Soap was made using coconut oil and wood ashes. But it was more than soap because it could be traded for much needed sugar. And that sugar was not only used to sweeten drinks and foods but can also be used to make alcohol for a fuel source to run automobile engines.

Fertig Coconut Oil: Coconut oil has many uses and one main use was for fuel to run the diesel generators to make electricity for radios, lights,... Fertig himself used coconut oil on his chapped lips.

If you go an any outdoor adventure, take a couple fresh coconuts with you - they'll make your outdoor adventure more enjoyable and could save your life Anytime Anywhere!

Coconut Survival: I'm telling you, you have to take coconuts on all your outdoor adventures cause they suffice the *8 Elements of Survival* (Fire, Water, Shelter, First-Aid, Signal, Food, Weapons and Navigation). I already told you plenty about coconut uses in the 2003, 2004, 2005, 2006, 2007 and in this Newsletter for more great "coconut" survival data so you're ready Anytime Anywhere.

And here's some more great news about them life-saving coconuts and it comes from 02 great magazines called Fit Yoga (February 2007 issue - writer Mara McFalls) and Woman's World Magazine (13 February 2007). Anyway, here's some more facts:

k) Genuine Coconut Oil Products: Here are a couple genuine coconut oil products you should know about. I've used them for years so there worthy of you looking into them. The 1st product is called Extra Virgin, Certified Coconut Oil. It's made by Emerals Laboratories and it has a few "uns" to it. Their product is Undeodorized, Unprocessed, Unrefined, Unheated, Raw, and Extra Virgin.

And there's a lot more healthy reasons to get their product as stated on the back label (Cholesterol Control, Immune System, Intestinal Health,...).

Another coconut oil product you ought to look into is called Organic Coconut Oil and it's made by Spectrum.

Important Note: When exposed to the sun and or air, coconut water loses its nutrients.

NG Dhow Maintenance: In the past 2,000 years, a variety of dhows (wooden ships) have sailed the Arab seas. And for centuries, the crew of these ships have improvised to protect themselves and their ships. Let's start with *Coconut Matting*.

a) Coconut Matting: Matting made from coconut fiber was woven to make mats. These large mats were stabilized vertically around the outer perimeter of the ship. The coconut mats protected the crew and cargo from sea water spray during rough seas.

b) Underwater Hull Protectant: The hulls of dhows were made of all wood. To protect the hull (below water level) from eating teredo worms and parasitic barnacles, a concoction of goat fat and lime is rubbed on the hull.

c) Above Water Hull Protectant: Again, the hulls of dhows were made of wood. To protect the hull (above water level) from decaying seawater, the hulls were rubbed with shark oil. Hulls protected by shark oil turned to a color of reddish brown. (NG = National Geographic - September 1974)

Coconut Update: Remember the LOST R&D from the 2004 Newsletter (Lost Coconut R & D! - Item 264 - Coconut Kindling on page 53)? Well here's an update. On 19 May 2003, I bagged thin slices of coconut meat. Here it is 02 April 2004 - almost 11-months later.

I retrieved a thin slice of coconut meat - it still looks white, no mold, no deterioration, and it's still edible - no I didn't drop dead from food poisoning. It did harden a bit more over the months but still held plenty of coconut oil.

I took a match to it and it still ignited and fired-up, complimented with its 4th of July type miniature fireworks of crackling, popping, spitting fire of different colors,... It burned with a very vigorous, 09-inch high orange flame with some black smoke and complimented with miniature fireworks for 03-mins & 15-secs.

Now you know, slices of coconut are not only long-lasting but are an edible food and great kindling for emergency fire-starting for at least 11-months while secured in a ziplock bag.

Bataan Sun Helmet: If Bataan Sun Helmet: The sun was a real whoopin' in itself. Some POWs that were caught trying to escape were stripped naked and pegged spread eagle to the ground where they were literally being baked by the hot shining sun. This was done in plain view of other POWs as an example. The baking POWs hurt so bad they were screaming to their Japanese captors to shoot them dead.

But the Japanese let them bake for several hours before they untied them, had them dig their own graves and executed them for all the POWs to witness under the sun. The sun was a sure killer and to shield them from it, POWs made sun helmets. POWs made sun helmets using coconut fiber. It was simple to make, very lightweight, provided ventilation, and most of all it shielded their heads from the deadly hot baking sun.

More Tasty Info On More Nuts You Should Know About For Vibrant Energy!

Here are a few other nuts and their facts and benefits you should know about. Let's start with *Hazel Nuts*.

a) HAZEL NUTS: Hazel nuts are also called filberts. Hazel nuts provide:

Vitamins---Vitamins B for energy. Vitamin E for healthy hair, nails, and skin. Vitamin fiber, good fats, minerals, protein, and vitamins.

Minerals---Minerals like calcium, magnesium, and potassium. **Calcium** is vital to your health. Ninety-nine (99) percent of all calcium is found in our bones. A lack of this very important nutrient can lead to loss of height, teeth, back pain, and weak porous bones that can crack or break. As your body matures, the demand for calcium increases. Magnesium relaxes the nerves and muscles. This mineral is known as the *"anti-stress"* mineral. Magnesium converts blood sugar into energy. This mineral helps keep teeth healthy and provides temporary relief from indigestion.

This mineral is necessary so that our body can use Vitamin C, calcium, phosphorus, sodium, and potassium effectively. Magnesium is essential in over 300 enzyme activities, especially the production of ATP (helps supply energy to every part of your body).

Magnesium is a must for healthy hearts! As a matter of fact, research has indicated multitudes of heart disease related deaths are linked to magnesium deficiency! **Potassium**, along with sodium, helps regulate the water balance within the body and transports nutrients. This mineral is also instrumental in helping send messages through our nervous system. The heart and other muscles are dependent on potassium for a healthy state and their proper function. Excessive salt, sugar, diuretics, laxatives, alcohol, and stress can deplete the body of this vital mineral.

Good Fats---Hazel nuts are loaded with polyunsaturated fats and monounsaturated fats. **Polyunsaturated fats** may lower the cholesterol in the blood. Other sources of polyunsaturated fats are corn, safflower, soybean and sunflower seed oils. **Monounsaturated fats** help maintain HDL (high density lipoprotein) that helps prevent heart disease. Olive oil, peanut oil, and canola oil are noted to be highest in monounsaturated fats.

Phytochemicals---Hazelnuts contains phytopchemicals to include proanthocyanidins, quercetin, and kaempherol. **Phytochemicals** are the natural chemical compounds found in all plants. Phytochemicals are naturally occurring chemicals in plants that give fruits, vegetables, grains and legumes their medicinal, disease-preventing, health enhancing properties. Phytochemicals are noted to be powerful antioxidant nutrients.

Proanthocyanidins, in the 1950's, Professor Jacques Masquelier of the University of Bordeaux, France isolated active components of the pine bark; they were found along the St. Lawrence River and other parts of the world. There are 20,000 different types of and combinations of bioflavonoids. One particular group is vastly superior because it is water-soluble and highly bioavailable. This group of bioflavonoids is called proanthocyanidins! The most powerful and health-enhancing and beneficial proanthocyanidins come from the bark of the maritime pine, Pinus maritima, growing along the southern coast of France from Bordeaux to the Spanish border. This bark contains the LARGEST AMOUNTS of the ACTIVE INGREDIENTS!

Also called of Pycnogenol (PROANTHOCYANIDINS), these special compounds allow the Bordeaux pine to withstand the harsh winds of winter, the blinding sun and intense heat of summer, and the salty winds of the Atlantic Ocean! Proanthocyanidins are non-toxic and are powerful heavyweights when it comes to antioxidants! Dubbed OPCs for short, they can be extracted from a few certain species of pine trees. OPCs have been extensively tested throughout the world for toxicity and have been concluded as being completely safe and non-toxic!

Quercetin is a yellow crystalline pigment present in plants, used as a food supplement to reduce allergic responses and / or boost immunity. <u>Are you one of millions of Americans that drip, sneeze, wheeze every spring, summer, and fall? Are you allergic to dust pollen and pets? Would you like to know how to remedy your allergy and asthma?</u> Quercetin, a bioflavonoid, may be the answer! Usually triggered by air or food-borne pollens and chemicals called allergens. These allergens are absorbed into your blood through your intestines, lungs, or skin.

These allergens cause B cells (white blood cells) of allergy sufferers to release billions of molecules of the allergic antibody IgE. These IgE molecules travel through your bloodstream until they combine with mast cells or basophils. Mast cells and basophils are main storage sites for histamine and serotonin. The IgE allergic antibody causes the mast cells and basophils to become *"leaky"* which unloads their storage sites of histamine and serotonin to pour into your blood and tissues. This produces the typical blocked sinuses, coughing, itchy eyes, runny nose, skin blotches, swollen nose, and wheezing. So where does Quercetin come into play? Quercetin has a strong attraction for both mast cells and basophils.

Quercetin is noted to stabilize their cell membranes, which prevents the mast cells and basophils from spilling their storage sites of histamine and serotonin into the surrounding blood and tissue in response to the initial IgE antibody in response to the allergen that penetrated your intestine, lungs, or skin in the first place! Asthma is an allergic inflammation involving your lungs. An asthma attack can be triggered by air or food-borne animal hair, chemicals, dust, or pollen. During an asthma attack, there are millions of tiny air sacs within your lungs that constrict and seriously impair breathing. You may feel a tightness in your chest. Besides the release of IgE-released histamine as mentioned above, the main cause of asthmatic symptoms is from a group of fatty acid derivatives called leukotrienes (LTs). Quercetin is noted to help prevent the forming of these asthma-causing LTs and you already know the roll it play against the release histamines.

Kaempferol was discovered in 1938 by the Hungarian biochemist Albert Szent-Györgyi as part of the flavonoid family. It's one of the many flavonols that can be found in plant based foods and is part of the phytonutrient family. It's a strong antioxidant to help prevent oxidative damage to cells and DNA. Protecting DNA from oxidative damage can also help protect against cancer, by preventing mutations from occurring in the first place. Lab studies have found that this natural compound inhibits the formation of cancer cells and their growth. It's been seen to be effective in combination with quercetin. Kaempferol also appears to make cancer cells more sensitive to anti-cancer agents, including chemotherapy drugs.

Besides a cancer-preventer & fighter, kaempferol acts ab an antioxidant, antidepressant, phytoestrogen (a compound which regulates estrogen levels in the body and can help prevent cancer, heart disease, osteoporosis (reduced bone mineral density) and negative menopausal symptoms), metabolism, preventing arteriosclerosis (hardening and loss of elasticity within the arteries), and helps prevent cancers including breast cancer, lung cancer, ovarian cancer, pancreatic cancer, and prostate cancer. Kaempferol can be found in foods and drinks including apples, black tea, blueberries, onions, oranges, turnip greens, red wine, and spinach. See *Kjoules Table – Energy Ratings For Nuts* in the next Section.

b) WALNUTS: Brazil Nut Tree (Bertholletia excelsa), native to northern Brazil. There are several species of walnuts but the most common species of walnuts are the English or Persian Walnut and the Black Walnut. Walnuts secret an ingredient into the soil to prevent other plants from growing near it. Upon ripening. the wrinkly round brown walnut shell forming 02 halves is secured in a green husk. Inside the shell are 02 kernels of meat loaded with antioxidants. The antioxidants help the oil-rich seed from oxygen which prevents rancidity. Freshly harvested walnuts are best stored in low humidity at temperatures of 27-degrees to 32-degrees Fahrenheit. Vacuum packing the walnut seeds at the recommended temperatures may be a good idea. Walnuts provide a BOUNTY of nutrients like carbohydrates, dietary fiber, saturated fats, monounsaturated fats, polyunsaturated fats, protein, vitamin A, beta-carotene, lutein zeaxanthin, thiamine (B1), riboflavin (B2), niacin (B3), pantothenic acid (B5) vitamin B6, folate (B9), vitamin B12, vitamin C, vitamin D, vitamin D, vitamin E, vitamin K, calcium, iron, magnesium, manganese, phosphorus, potassium, sodium, and zinc. See *Kjoules Table - Energy Ratings For Nuts* in the next Section.

c) MACADAMIA NUTS: Macadamia nuts are indigenous to Australia. Delicious macadamia nuts are loaded with tasty fats. Of the few species of macadamia nuts, only 02 species (Macadamia integrifolia and Macadamia tetraphylla) can be eaten raw. Macadamia nuts are loaded with carbohydrates, fiber, fats (saturated fats, monounsaturated fats, polyunsaturated fats), protein, vitamins like thiamine (B1), riboflavin (B2), niacin (B3), pantothenic acid (B5), vitamin B6, folate (B9), vitamin C, vitamin E, minerals like calcium, iron, magnesium, manganese, phosphorus, potassium, and zinc.

WARNING: Macadamia nuts are toxic to dogs. The consumption of macadamia nuts by dogs could bring on weakness with hind limb paralysis, unable to stand, muscle tremors, joint pain, severe abdominal pain,…

Cosmetics containing macadamia oil may cause allergic reactions to users applying it as a makeup product. See *Kjoules Table - Energy Ratings For Nuts* in the next Section.

d) PINE NUTS: There are about 20 species of tasty pine nuts throughout the world that are harvested for consumption. I myself was brought up and raised on harvesting and eating pine nuts. I remember one time we (family members) harvested a military duffle bag full of pine nuts. We took the shelled pine nut and roasted them in the oven. They were delicious plus you can eat them raw. Delicious pine nuts are loaded with tasty fat and other nutrients. Nutrients like: starch, sugars, dietary fiber, saturated fat, monounsaturated fat, polyunsaturated fat, protein, vitamin A equivalent beta-carotene, thiamine (B1), riboflavin (B2), niacin (B3), pantothenic acid (B5), vitamin B6, folate (B9), choline, vitamin C, vitamin E, vitamin K, calcium, iron, magnesium, manganese, phosphorus, potassium, and zinc.

One most important facts I want to annotate here is the calorie food energy is measured in joules. The nutritional value of pines nuts per 100 grams or 03.5 ounces is equal to 2,815 kJ (673 kcal). Which brings me again to the Donner Party.

"The Forlorn Hope weakly continued on. They were so weak, to just step over a downed log, they had to roll over it! The last few days they came across a few Indian tribes and they didn't care if they were hostile or not. Some tribes felt pity for the ragged group and did in fact help them with navigation, and food (raw acorns, prepared acorn meal loafs - November 2000 Newsletter).

On 17 January, the chief of one Indian village gave Eddy a handful of pine nuts! After eating them, Eddy "felt wonderfully refreshed!" See Kjoules Table - Energy Ratings For Nuts in the next Section.

e) CHESTNUTS: Native American Indians were eating chestnuts – namely the American chestnuts long before Europeans brought European chestnuts to North America. For example chestnuts found in the Appalachian Mountains accounted for 25% of the hardwood trees found in these mountains. For about 300-years, most barns and homes were constructed using chestnut wood. And those chestnuts from the tall 50 – 100-foot trees, fall to the ground are easily retrieved. Chestnuts are roasted and also made into many different recipes. Chestnuts provide sugars, fat, protein, vitamin A equiv., thiamine (B1), riboflavin (B2), niacin (B3), vitamin B6, folate (B9), vitamin B12, vitamin C, calcium, iron, magnesium, phosphorus, potassium, sodium, and zinc. So go get you a batch of chestnuts and *'roast em' over an open fire.'* See *Kjoules Table - Energy Ratings For Nuts* in the next Section.

f) CASHEW NUTS: I think salted cashews are the tastiest of all the several types of nuts I listed in this book. Originally from Brazil, the cashew is also harvested (Top 05 countries) in Benin (West Africa), Côte d'Ivoire (West Africa), India, Nigeria, Vietnam, Nigeria, with a total production of 4,439,960 metric tons with Vietnam harvesting the most cashews at 1,110,800 metric tons.

The cashew tree (Anacardium occidentale) is a tropical evergreen tree that produces the cashew seed and the cashew apple. The cashew nut is actually not a nut but a seed. The cashew tree grows as high as 46-feet. The dwarf cashew tree grows up to 20-feet high and is harvested more than the taller cashew tree because it matures earlier and produces more cashew seeds (nuts). The mature cashew can be eaten raw and is prepared worldwide in various meals, deserts, and drinks. See *Kjoules Table - Energy Ratings For Nuts* in the next Section.

g) PECAN NUTS: The pecan is a very large deciduous (leaves fall off every Fall season) tree that can reach a height of 144-feet with a trunk as wide as 06 1/2-feet in diameter. Pecan trees can produce pecans for up to 300 years. The seeds (nuts) of the pecan can be eaten as is or roasted and prepared for desserts and candies. The pecan delivers a tasty buttery flavor. The USA harvests the most pecans (200,000 tons) worldwide with the state of Georgia the top producer See *Kjoules Table - Energy Ratings For Nuts* in the next Section.

h) PISTACHIO NUTS: It's no wonder the pistachio seed (nut) is very tasty because it's part of the cashew family and the small tree originated from Central Asia and the Middle East. Archeologist discovered that pistachios were a common food as far back as 6,750 B.C. (Before Christ).

The pistachio is highly tolerant to saline soil because it is a desert plant. And it's a durable plant and can withstand temperatures down to 14-degrees Fahrenheit and up to 118-degrees Fahrenheit. An average pistachio tree provides 50,000 seeds every 02-years. And the seeds are protected beige-colored shell. The shell naturally splits open when its ready to be harvested.

Approximately 916,921 metric tons of pistachios are harvested each year with Iran on top of the list with 478,600 metric tons with the US of A coming in second with 196,930 metric tons with Turkey, China, and Syria the other top harvesters. China consumes the most pistachios with a consumption total of 80,000 tons with the US of A coming in second with a total consumption of 45,000 tons. Pistachios provides carbohydrates, fiber, saturated fat, monounsaturated fats, polyunsaturated fats, protein, vitamin A equiv. - lutein zeaxanthin, thiamine (B1), riboflavin (B2), niacin (B3), pantothenic acid (B5), vitamin B6, folate (B9), vitamin B12, vitamin C, vitamin D, vitamin E, calcium, iron, magnesium, manganese, phosphorus, potassium, and zinc. See *Kjoules Table - Energy Ratings For Nuts* in the next Section.

WARNING: If the pistachio seeds are contaminated with mold, aflatoxin may be the result. Aflatoxin are powerful carcinogenic (cancer causing) ingredients. So never eat any pistachios or any food that's contaminated with mold. There is an exception but that's another subject (*Healing Mold* - 2005 Anytime Anywhere Survival Newsletter [AASN]).

i) ALMOND NUTS: The almond tree is a deciduous tree and grows as high as 33-feet and grows best in Mediterranean climates of the Middle East with warm dry summers and mild wet winters. Almonds are grown in several countries to include Afghanistan, Australia, India, Iran, Morocco, Pakistan, Spain, United States (California), with the USA producing 01.8 million tonnes of the almost 03 million tonnes produced worldwide. Three years after its planted it will start bearing almonds and between 05 to 07 years it reaches its full bearing capacity and in the Fall months the almonds reach maturity for harvesting.

Almond nuts provide a bounty of nutrients especially in the department of protein. It provides starch, sugars lactose, dietary fiber, saturated fats, monounsaturated fats, polyunsaturated fats, tryptophan, threonine, isoleucine, leucine, lysine, methionine, cystine, phenylalanine, tyrosine, valine, arginine, histidine, alanine, aspartic acid, glutamic acid, glycine, proline, serine, vitamin A equiv. beta-carotene, lutein zeaxanthin, vitamin A 1 iu, thiamine (B1), riboflavin (B2), niacin (B3), pantothenic acid (B5), vitamin B6, folate (B9), choline, vitamin C, vitamin D, vitamin E, vitamin K, calcium, iron, magnesium, manganese, phosphorus, potassium, sodium, and zinc. See *Kjoules Table - Energy Ratings For Nuts* in the next Section.

j) SOY NUTS: Soy nuts are actually made from soybeans that are soaked in water, drained, and then they're baked or roasted. Soy nuts are high in protein (all essential amino acids) and dietary fiber. Soy nuts is a dense food meaning there are a lot of nutrients and fat content packed in a small serving. Only 01 or 02-ounces of soy nuts are recommended per day. Just ¼-cup of soy nuts provide plenty of protein, carbohydrates, vitamins (B-1, B-2, B-6, and K), fiber, minerals (iron, magnesium, phosphorus, potassium, and zinc) and fat (saturated fat, monounsaturated, polyunsaturated fats to include omega-3 fatty acids and omega-6 fatty acids). Soy nut also provide isoflavones. Isoflavones are compounds similar to the hormone estrogen (female sex hormone). A combination of isoflavones and <u>soy</u> protein helps to lower LDL cholesterol (bad cholesterol). Isoflavones also help to avoid cognitive decline. Isoflavones also aid in bone formation and help prevent osteoporosis (bones become weak and brittle). See *Kjoules Table - Energy Ratings For Nuts* in the next Section.

Not: If soy nuts are roasted, approximately 50% of protein (amino acids) is lost.

k) Pili Nuts: The pili tree grows up to 66-feet tall and is a tropical tree native to Southeast Asia, Papua New Guinea, and Northern Australia. Pili nuts are harvested in the Philippines.

The brownish pili nut is composed of approximately 70% fat, 08% carbohydrates, up to 13.9% protein and 16% cotyledons (seed leaf). The raw pili nut tastes like a roasted pumpkin seed. And when it's roasted it has a mild nutty flavor and feel it has a taste superior to the almond nut. The pili nut is used to make cakes, chocolate, ice cream, and other baked goods. The pili nut is loaded with fats, protein, manganese, calcium, phosphorus, and potassium. See *Kjoules Table - Energy Ratings For Nuts* in the next Section.

m) Eastern Black Walnuts: The Eastern Black Walnut is native to North America. The black walnut tree can grow as high as 131-feet and can be found as far west to South Dakota, southwest to central Texas and as far south to northern Florida. The walnut fruit including the husk falls to the ground in the Fall months. Popular uses of the black walnut are bakery goods, chicken, cookies, fish, fudge, ice cream, pasta dishes, pies, pork, salads, vegetables,… In the Spring time, the black walnut tree can be tapped for a sweet sap that can be drunk as is or concentrated into a syrup or sugar.

Tapped in spring, the tree yields a sweet sap that can be drunk or concentrated into syrup or sugar.[citation needed]

Black walnuts provide carbohydrates, starch, sugars, dietary fiber, saturated fat, monounsaturated fat, polyunsaturated omega-3, omega-6, protein, vitamin A, thiamine (B1), riboflavin (B2), niacin (B3), pantothenic acid (B5), vitamin B6, folate (B9), vitamin B12, vitamin C, vitamin D, vitamin E, vitamin K, calcium, iron, magnesium, manganese, phosphorus, potassium, sodium, and zinc. See *Kjoules Table - Energy Ratings For Nuts* in the next Section.

n) SUNFLOWER SEEDS: Sunflower seeds are a popular healthfood snack. And they're used to enhance the taste for many recipes like salads, candies, breads, soups, energy bars, energy drinks,… Bags of <u>shelled sunflower seeds</u> can be purchased in most stores and are so popular, they come with different flavors like Regular Salted, Regular Unsalted, Ranch, BBQ, Smoky BBQ, Dill Pickle, Cracked Pepper, Black Pepper, Bacon, Buffalo Wing, Jalapeño, Spicy Garlic, Salt & Pepper, Bacon Ranch, Buffalo Style Ranch, Nacho Cheese, Bloody Mary, Green Chili,… Sunflower seeds are also put in pet foods and used in bird feeders. And sunflower oil has become popular and mostly used for cooking. Sunflower seeds provide carbohydrates, sugars, dietary fiber, saturated fat, monounsaturated fat, polyunsaturated fat, protein, thiamine (B1), riboflavin (B2), niacin (B3), pantothenic acid (B5), vitamin B6, folate (B9), choline, vitamin C, vitamin E, calcium, iron, magnesium, manganese, phosphorus, potassium, sodium, and zinc. See *Kjoules Table - Energy Ratings For Nuts* in the next Section.

Kjoules Table - Energy Ratings For Nuts!

Here are the Kjoules Ratings for the following nuts. This translate into how much energy per the amount of calories that particular nut is providing for you – thus the energy measured in joules. The higher the Kjoules Rating the more energy it will provide for you. Pick out your favorite tasty nuts with its Kjoules Rating so you're super energetic Anytime Anywhere! OK, let's get started.

Coconut----------------100 grams or 03.5 ounces is equal to 354 kcal (1,480 kJ)

Cashew Nuts----------100 grams or 03.5 ounces is equal to 553 kcal (2,310 kJ)

Chestnuts--------------100 grams or 03.5 ounces is equal to 820 kJ (200 kcal)

Raisins-----------------100 grams or 03.5 ounces is equal to 1,252 kJ (299 kcal)

Soy Nuts---------------100 grams or 03.5 ounces is equal to 1,866 kJ (446 kcal)

Pistachio Nuts--------100 grams or 03.5 ounces is equal to 2,351 kJ (562 kcal)

Peanuts-----------------100 grams or 03.5 ounces is equal to 2,385 kJ (570 kcal)

Pumpkin Seeds-------100 grams or 03.5 ounces is equal to 2,401 kJ (574 kcal)

Almond Nuts----------100 grams or 03.5 ounces is equal to 2,408 kJ (576 kcal)

Sunflower Seeds------100 grams or 03.5 ounces is equal to 2,445 kJ (584 kcal)

Peanut Butter----------100 grams or 03.5 ounces is equal to 2,462 kJ (588 kcal)

Black Walnut----------100 grams or 03.5 ounces is equal to 2,586 kJ (618 kcal)

Hazelnuts---------------100 grams or 03.5 ounces is equal to 2,629 kJ (628 kcal)

Walnut------------------100 grams or 03.5 ounces is equal to 2,738 kJ (654 kcal)

Brazil Nuts-------------100 grams or 03.5 ounces is equal to 2,743 kJ (656 kcal)

Pine Nuts---------------100 grams or 03.5 ounces is equal to 2,815 kJ (673 kcal)

Pecan Nuts-------------100 grams or 03.5 ounces is equal to 2,889 kJ (690 kcal)

Pili Nuts----------------100 grams or 03.5 ounces is equal to 3,008 kJ (719 kcal)

Macadamia Nuts-----100 grams or 03.5 ounces is equal to 3,080 kJ (740 kcal)

Cal = Calories

J = Joules

K = 1,000

MOST IMPORTANT NOTE: You already read my take on Trail-Mix. If you decide to make your own trail-mix for your next outdoor adventure, consider the nuts with the highest joule ratings so your trail-mix is LOADED with energy-producing foods. Also let your tastebuds help you decide what kind of trail-mix you want to make. You may also want to add a pinch of sea salt to each pack cause you're gonna need the sodium in your system when venturing outdoors. And don't forget, those nuts are loaded with oil for emergency fire-stating. For example the Brazil nut. That baby has an average burn time of 06-minutes and 36-seconds. One last thing, once you make your own separate packs trail-mix, INSURE you pack it so it's absolutely water-tight. Try to vacuum pack each pack, then wrap it up again and mark it (all ingredients), date produced, and Expiration Date.

Power Bar Recipe!

Here's a tasty Power Bar recipe so you can really be ENERGIZED Anytime Anywhere - plus you can save a bunch of money by making them yourself cause Power Bars cost between $1 to $2 each!

Ingredients: To make Power Bars, you'll need the following ingredients. One baking sheet (10-inch by 15-inch), one can of non-stick cooking spray, large bowl, two eggs, two cups of all-purpose flour, two sticks of butter, one and one-half of cups of rolled oats, one cup of white sugar, one-half cup of brown sugar, one teaspoon of vanilla extract, one teaspoon of salt, one teaspoon of baking soda, one cup of dried cranberries, and one cup of chopped pecans.

Step 01: Preheat your oven to 375-degrees. Coat the baking sheet with non-stick cooking spray.

Step 02: Place the butter, both white & brown sugars, eggs and vanilla extract in the large bowl and stir to a creamy consistency.

Step 03: Add the flour, salt, baking soda, and oats in the large bowl and mix well.

Step 04: Add the cranberries and pecans and stir.

Step 05: Place the concoction on the baking sheet and spread evenly.

Step 06: Bake for 20 to 25 minutes.

Step 07: Test by placing a single toothpick in the concoction and pull-out. If it comes out clean, the Power Bars are done.

Step 08: Remove from oven and allow to cool.

Step 09: Cut Power Bars to your dimensions and place in sandwich bags for future use.

1st Note: You can also use other tasty ingredients like peanuts, walnuts, raisins, dried cherries, dried pineapple bits, dried peach bits,...

2nd Note: Power Bars cost about $2 bucks a shot! You can SAVE a lot of money by making your own tasty, nutritious Power Bars!

Points Of Contact!

10 Cool Facts About Coconuts (YouTube)-----https://youtu.be/o2AlPPKzY18

10 Surprising Facts About
The Largest Nut In The World--------------------http://www.agrana.com/en/products/fruit/fruit-preparations/trendblog/
fruit-of-the-month/coconut-fun-facts/

Coconut Facts for Kids----------------------------http://www.sciencekids.co.nz/sciencefacts/
food/coconuts.html

Coconut Nutrition----------------------------------http://www.cookycoconuts.com

Coconut Oil: 10 Fun Facts
About This Healthy Fat----------------------------http://bodyunburdened.com/
health-benefits-of-coconut-oil/

Coconut Research Center--------------------------http://www.coconutresearchcenter.org/

Coconut Secrets for Optimal Health--------------https://www.coconutsecret.com/
coconuthealthsecrets2.html

Coconut Tree Facts-------------------------------http://www.softschools.com/facts/
plants/coconut_tree_facts/560/

Coconut Uses Infographic-------------------------http://www.mercola.com/infographics/
coconut-uses.htm

Coconut Water Nutrition Facts--------------------http://www.nutrition-and-you.com/
coconut-water.html

Tropical Traditions----------------------------------http://www.tropicaltraditions.com
Offers high quality virgin coconut oil that is not processed and tainted like most inferior coconut oils.

More Survival Kindle E-Books And Survival Paperback Books For YOU!

Joseph A. Laydon Jr. (MSG Ret. Army) is the author and owner of Intensive Research Information Services And Products (IRISAP). Joseph has been writing "self-reliance" orientated data since 1991 and since July 2012 has been re-publishing his works via Kindle E-Books and CreateSpace Paperback Books. He has self-published more than **80+ Survival Books** (Kindle E-Books and Paperback Books). Below is a list of all his Survival Books and you can see these books by simply going to the 02 websites listed below for detailed descriptions and videos. See *"About Author."*

- **Kindle E-Books:**--------------------**www.survivalexpertebooks.com**

- **Paperback Books:**-----------------**www.survivalexpertbooks.com**

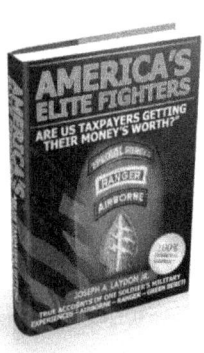 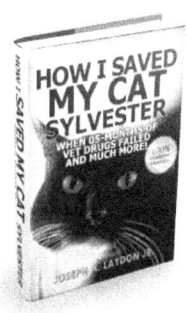 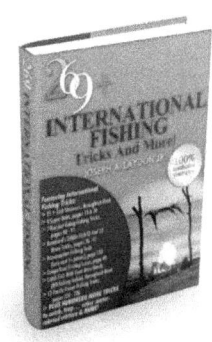

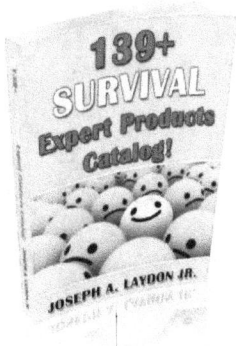

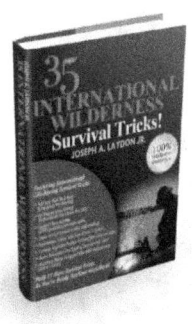

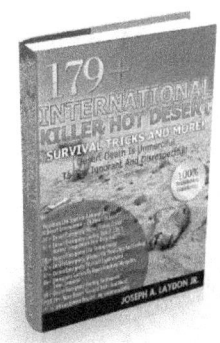

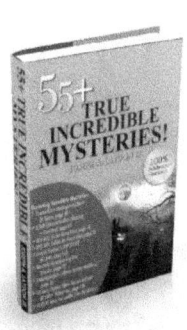

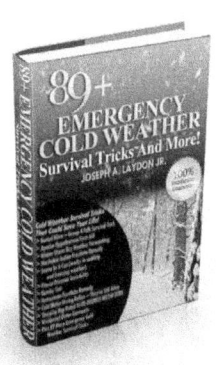

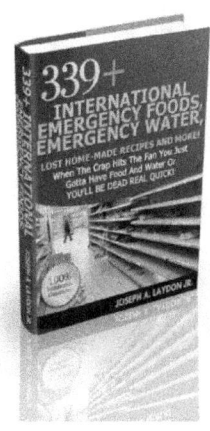

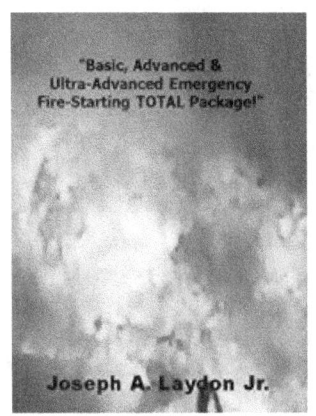

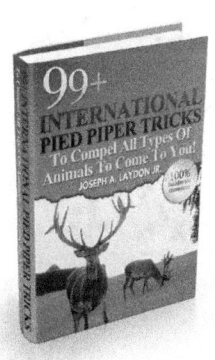

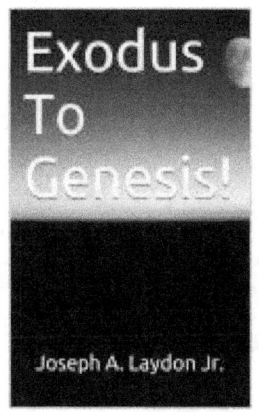

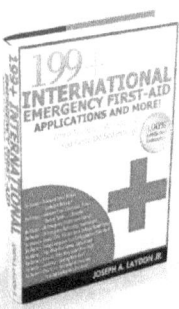

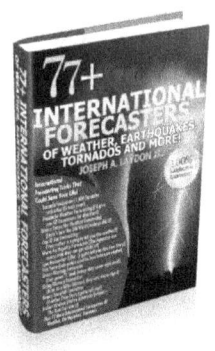

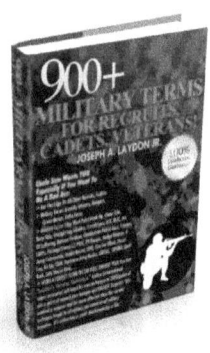

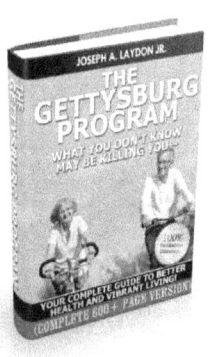

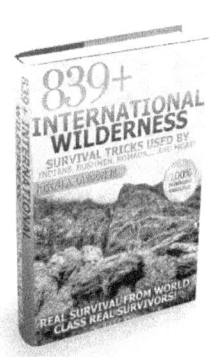

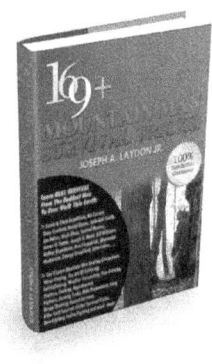

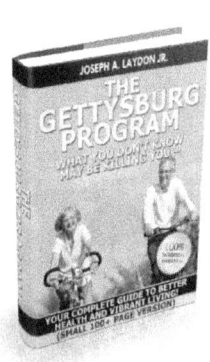

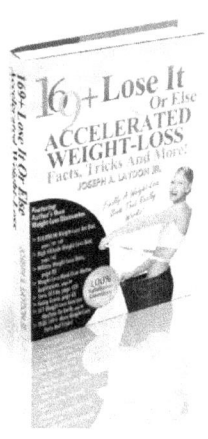

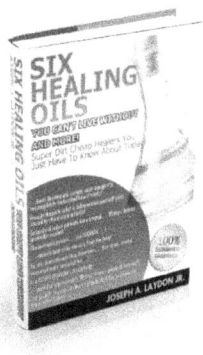

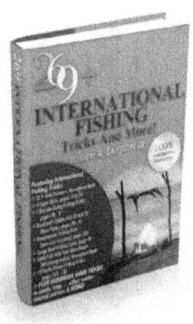

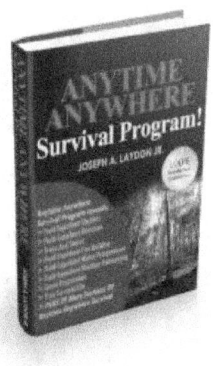

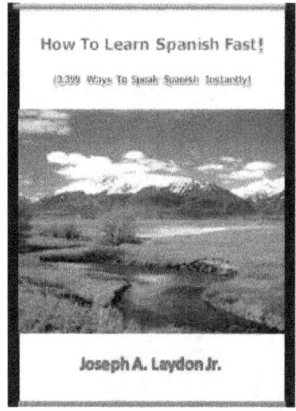

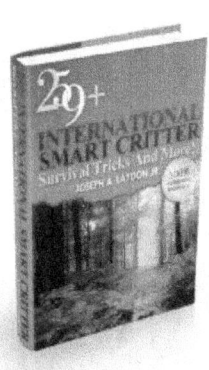

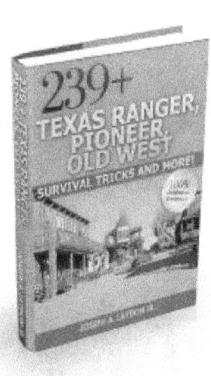

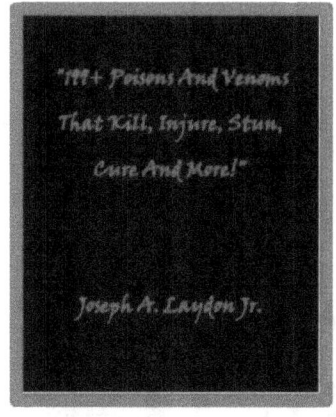

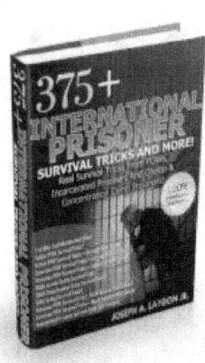

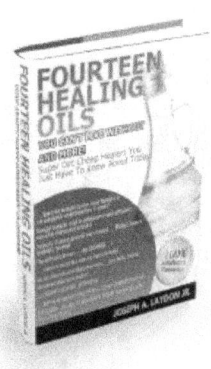

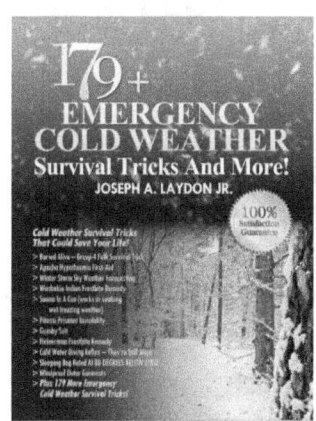

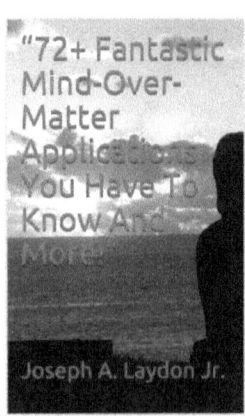

"72+ Fantastic Mind-Over-Matter Applications You Have To Know And More!"

Joseph A. Laydon Jr.

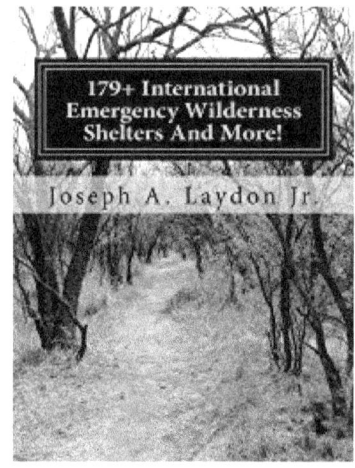

179+ International Emergency Wilderness Shelters And More!

Joseph A. Laydon Jr.

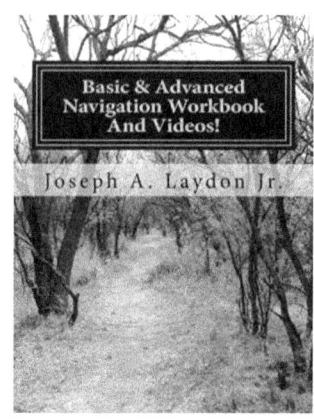

Basic & Advanced Navigation Workbook And Videos!

Joseph A. Laydon Jr.

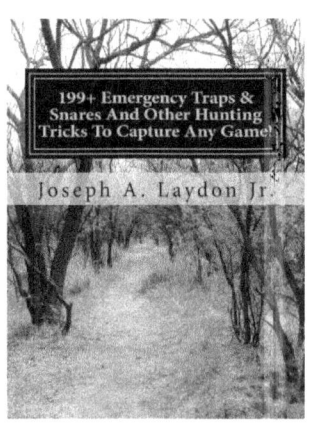

199+ Emergency Traps & Snares And Other Hunting Tricks To Capture Any Game!

Joseph A. Laydon Jr.

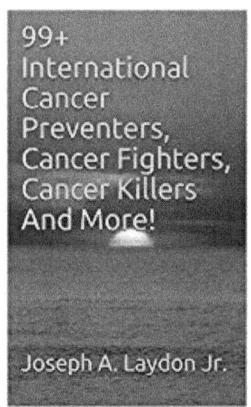

99+ International Cancer Preventers, Cancer Fighters, Cancer Killers And More!

Joseph A. Laydon Jr.

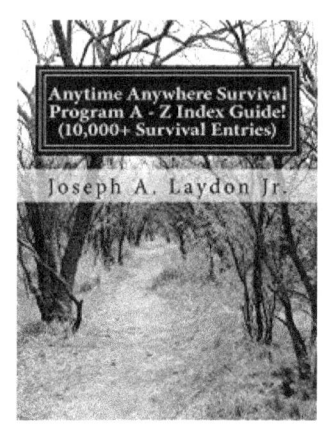

Anytime Anywhere Survival Program A - Z Index Guide! (10,000+ Survival Entries)

Joseph A. Laydon Jr.

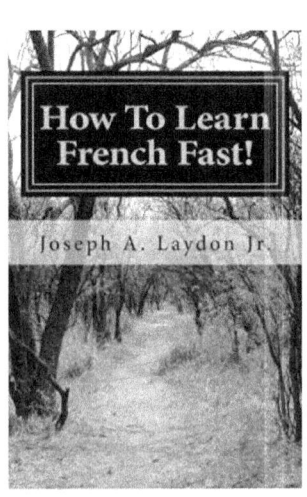

How To Learn French Fast!

Joseph A. Laydon Jr.

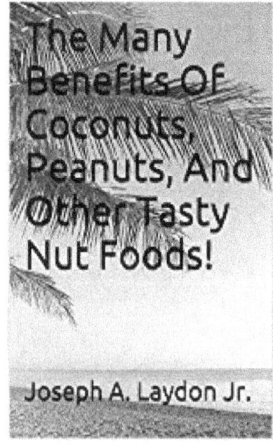

The Many Benefits Of Coconuts, Peanuts, And Other Tasty Nut Foods!

Joseph A. Laydon Jr.

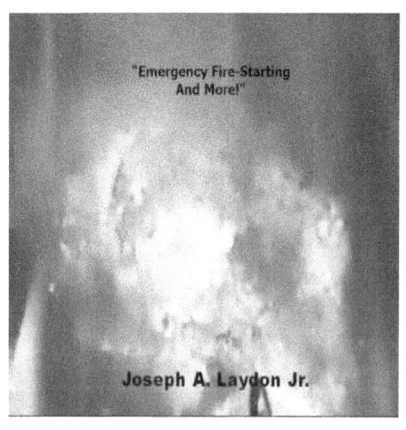

"Emergency Fire-Starting And More!"

Joseph A. Laydon Jr.

About The Author

Joseph A. Laydon Jr. (MSG Ret. Army - 18Z5V) is the author and owner of *Intensive Research Information Services And Products (IRISAP)*.

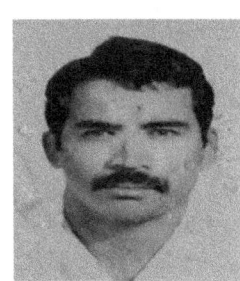

Joseph is a well-qualified instructor in international wilderness survival and the other 03 Survivals he teaches (Health, Crime, and Money). He is a 20-year US Army veteran (Master Sergeant E-8 - 18Z5V) associated with all Special Operations units in the US military, as well as Special Ops units in the Mid-East and Central & South America.

He's a qualified SERE Instructor (Survival Evasion Resistance & Escape) and has **taught wilderness survival** at the college level for 03 years. He's a qualified instructor in basic & advanced pistol marksmanship, basic & advanced rifle marksmanship, CQB (Close Quarter Battle), basic & advanced cross-country navigation, basic mountaineering techniques, and self-defense. Since 1994, he's published many self-improvement Survival Programs, Survival Videos, SPECIAL Reports, Intelligence Reports, monthly Newsletters, **80+ Survival Books** (Kindle E-Books & CreateSpace Paperback Books) and more in the works.

He's an inventor, he *"sideways engineers"* new survival tricks that can SAVE YOUR LIFE! An example: On 17 August 2000 - 1417 hours, at Scott Lake, Scott AFB, IL, Joseph made international history! He is the 1st in the world to replicate the mysterious fires of Africa using a single drop of water! On 05 January 2001, he discovered how to start a life-saving fire in just 02-seconds using a beam of light from a flashlight in pitch black *"blind man"* darkness! On 06 April 2005 - 1810 hours, he invented delicious & tasty Solid Fuel Rolls and several Trail-Mix Cookies that are used as emergency foods and used as long-burning emergency fire-starting kindling.

And recently - **50+ MORE TOP SECRET INVENTIONS** of advanced & ultra-advanced fire-starting like starting EMERGENCY FIRE-STARTING using personal care products and first-aid products you already use like:

- Shampoo
- Toothpastes
- Mouthwashes
- Breath Drops & Breath Sprays
- Salves
- Ointments
- Over-The-Counter Medicines
- Drink Enhancement Products
- Other ingredients like your spit (saliva), your urination,...

See **www.survivalexpert.com/fire**

He also teaches Advanced Navigation (*Basic & Advanced Navigation Workbook And Videos* [includes Workbook, Videos, maps, protractors,…]) so you're ready Anytime Anywhere! Only from IRISAP and only for privileged IRISAP subscribers - YOU! See *Basic & Advanced Navigation Workbook And Videos* at

www.survivalexpertbooks.com/navigation

Below is a sample of his military achievements & qualifications (<u>**not in chronological order**</u>) which reflect his unique & superior ability to teach basic, advanced & ultra-advanced survival applications, techniques and "tricks" that could help you AVOID serious killer survival threats as well as SAVE YOUR LIFE when you get in life or death situations. His trade secrets, Programs, and Videos are only offered to IRISAP subscribers-YOU!

- US Army Airborne School
- US Army Special Forces Qualification Course - SFQC (Green Beret)
- US Army Master Parachutist Wings
- Uruguayan Parachutist Wings
- British Parachutist Wings
- Kingdom of Jordan Parachutist Wings
- Expert Infantry Badge - EIB
- 82nd Airborne Division Recondo Course
- Adverse Weather Aerial Delivery System Tests - AWADS (01 of 386 volunteer paratroopers)
- US Army Special Forces Weapons Course (US & foreign pistols, submachineguns, assault rifles, rifles, machineguns, mortars, anti-tank weapons, anti-aircraft weapons,…)
- Weapons Armorer Course
- Indirect Fire Course (60mm, 81mm, & 4.2 inch *"four deuce"* mortars)
- Jumpmaster Course
- Basic French Language Course
- Combat Infantry Badge - CIB
- US Army Ranger Course
- Advanced Navigation Course
- Special Forces Sniper Course (02)
- Survival Evasion Resistance and Escape Instructor Course (SERE Level B)
- Wilderness Survival Instructor (College level - 03 years / 1991 - 1994)
- Rappell Master
- Fast Rope Master
- International Sniper Instructor
- International Close Quarter Battle (CQB) Instructor
- Participated In Multiple Combat Actions

- Special Forces Operations And Intelligence Course (O&I)
- Good Conduct Medal (06)
- Army Commendation Medal
- Army Achievement Medal (02)
- Meritorious Service Medal (02)
- Armed Forces Expeditionary Medal
- Letters Of Commendation (13)
- Letters Of Appreciation (08)
- Held **SECRET and TOP SECRET Clearances** for 20+ years

Featured on FOX-2 (24 August 2000). Joseph now resides in Illinois. He offers products concerning Wilderness Survival, Health Survival, Crime Survival, and Money Survival so to greatly enhance the lives of all IRISAP subscribers - YOU! Any questions, write to Joseph today.

Sincerely,
Joseph A. Laydon Jr. (IRISAP)
P.O. Box 48
Cutler, IL 62238-0048

You And Yours Have A Safe One
Anytime Anywhere,

Joseph A. Laydon Jr.

E-Mail: wwwsurvivalexpert@yahoo.com

WEBSITES
- Main Website--------------------------------www.survivalexpert.com
- 40+ Survival Paperback Books------------www.survivalexpertbooks.com
- 40+ Survival Kindle E-Books------------www.survivalexpertebooks.com
- Anytime Anywhere Survival--------------www.anytimeanywheresurvival.com
- Weight-Loss----------------------------www.loseitorelseweightloss.com
- True Scary Videos (all FREE)-----------www.truescaryvideos.com
- Exodus To Genesis----------------------www.exodustogenesis.com

Take Notes

Take Notes

Take Notes

Take Notes

Take Notes

Take Notes

Take Notes

Take Notes

"Survival Expert Private Mailing List!"

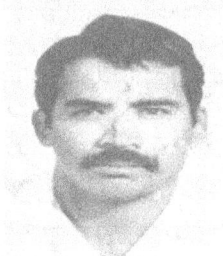

THANK YOU for your wise interest in this Survival Book. I have 80+ more Survival Books (Paperback Books & Kindle E-Books) that I've written and can be found at www.amazon.com See **www.survivalexpertbooks.com** and **www.survivalexpertebooks.com** for descriptions and videos on my books. And yes, I wrote every single word of each Survival Book. See *About The Author*.

Now let's get to my mailing list. How would you like get on my private 'Survival Expert' mailing list? NO, this isn't an e-mail list offer. This is a real – in your hands mailing list via the good ol' United States Postal Service.

I will cover the following subjects for each monthly mail-out:

- **Wilderness Survival**: I have THOUSANDS and THOUSANDS of real international survival tricks from the REAL SURVIVORS throughout the world and throughout history. Forget that worthless – 'will get you killed' - survival crap on television.

- **Health Survival**: I started my Health Survival back in the late 1990s. I study the stuff like I'm going to college. But I focus on dozens and dozens of Alternative Therapies. Here, let me tell you something that happened to me a couple years ago. A doctor in Sparta, IL told me 04-times, 04-times – quote: *"You have three weeks to live."* Hey, I'm still here. I'll tell you all about it PLUS a ton more of REAL Health Survival that's worthy of your attention for a healthy vibrant life.

- **Crime Survival**: Hey, you can be a bad ass in the woods and healthy as a horse but what about all those pieces of sh!+ cowards out there that will steal your money, hurt you, kill you or hurt & kill your loved ones in your home. I'll give you the Facts Of Life when it comes to Crime Survival and how to AVOID it and / or remedy it.

- **Money Survival**: We can all use more cash but I gotta tell you, most (95%) of that 'Make Money From Home' – excuse my language, is pure Bull Shit. They're all scams run by scumbags. And the few that are legit, it's still worthless. Why? Cause they can't teach. They just confuse and frustrate you till you give up. Now here's where I come in. I make some money via the internet. But most of my stuff on the internet are like Business Cards. People go to my several websites to check out that I'm a real person and they can see that I really do have my own Survival Products.

If you're interested in starting / re-starting your own home-based business and learning some super simple & unique applications that I use all the time and you're interested in the other Survivals - Wilderness Survival, Health Survival and Crime Survival, read my FREE OFFER. On the next few pages is my **FREE OFFER** for YOU. **DON'T SEND ME ANY MONEY**. Check out my **FREE OFFER** below.

"DO NOT SEND ME ANY MONEY. I Will Send You Any 03 Of 10 Survival Tricks Of Your Choice At NO-CHARGE!"

WILDERNESS-SURVIVAL   HEALTH-SURVIVAL   CRIME-SURVIVAL   MONEY-SURVIVAL

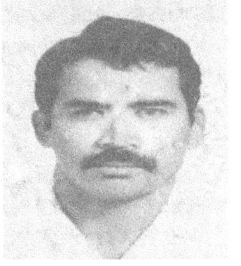

Hello, my name is Joseph A. Laydon Jr. (Cutler, IL). Since 1991 I've been teaching good folks like you REAL international survival. I have very satisfied customers from Canada to South Africa.

I will send you **any 03 international survival tricks of your choice** that you can use to AVOID trouble in the first place and get you out of trouble when your life and the lives of your loved ones are on the line.

Here's a quick list of all 10 Survival Tricks so You're Ready Anytime Anywhere. Somebody has to be the hero, why not YOU! OK, here's the list:

- PRSC
- Sauna In A Can!
- Home Invasion Defense!
- Laydon's Burn Remedy!
- Snakebite & Brown Recluse Spider Bite Remedy!
- Starting An Emergency Fire – Rub Your Shoe On A Rock!
- Panamanian Fishing Trick (100 Fish)!
- 100% Accurate Weather Forecasting Trick!
- Goose Final Approach!
- No Weapon Duck Hunting!

Private Message & Bonus
www.survivalexpertbooks.com/
private-list
(Special Bonus Just For YOU)

Now here are the descriptions for each of the 10 survival tricks. I will send you any 03 survival tricks of your choice - FREE – AT NO CHARGE!

Why? Cause once you see the great quality of the survival tricks you pick, I know you'll want all the others listed here PLUS 100 more for the small cost of a double cheeseburger, large fries and large coke. I'll send you 100+ more survival tricks so You're Ready Anytime Anywhere! OK, let's get started with the 10 international survival tricks. I'll send you any 03 of your choice FREE At NO-CHARGE! Let's start with *PRSC*.

01) PRSC!: I've had customers thank me for sending them *PRSC*. One customer wrote me and asked if I knew **how many lives I've saved with PRSC**.

PRSC is an acronym used by US Army Infantry units during their planning for combat missions. *PRSC* is used to keep soldiers from getting killed. I 'civilianized' *PRSC* for you and I have been teaching *PRSC* since the mid-1990s. *PRSC* could SAVE YOUR LIFE and the lives under your care.

I hear about outdoor tragedies (deaths) happening all the time and I nod my head thinking '*if they used PRSC*' or was one of my subscribers, **they'd be alive today**.' I'll tell you all about *PRSC* once you give me your go ahead to send you **any 03 survival tricks of your choice!**

02) Sauna In A Can!: I entered the US Army and was in the Infantry assigned to the 82nd Airborne out of Fort Bragg, NC. I gotta tell you, Airborne Infantry is a miserable miserable job and on top of that we jumped out of C-130 aircraft at 1 o'clock in the morning loaded down with all kinds of gear, severely nauseated and we were always cold and soaking wet. Back then, there was no fancy Goretex to keep us dry.

Well during a 03-week Recondo School I was attending, I was assigned Assistant Patrol Leader. We were out in the woods in the dead of winter learning patrolling. That North Carolina cold is a wet cold, a humid cold and it goes right thru you – it stings, it hurts. Anyway, I was going around the perimeter making sure the patrol members weren't sleeping. Everybody was cold and miserable in our foxholes. But one Private kept smiling up at me every time I passed by his foxhole.

Finally I whispered something like 'what is wrong with you?

Why aren't you miserable like the rest of us?' He then told me he was toasty warm and what he was doing and after I graduated from that course, I started using it too and used it throughout my military career. I nicknamed it *Sauna In A Can.* And it works even if you're shivering soaking wet and you're freezing to death! How does it work? I'll tell you EVERYTHING once I get your OK to send you **any 03 survival tricks!**

03) Home Invasion Defense!: Between 2003 and 2007, an estimated 3,700,000 homes were burglarized on average in the US. And about 28% of the time, home owners were present during the burglary. The term home invasion has been broadened to other home crimes besides simple burglary. **Before I carry-on, read that folded-up page attached to this letter.**

You'll see that I was an international sniper instructor and an international Close Quarter Battle (CQB) instructor. I took part in many many high risk and challenging training exercises and combat missions. I always thought the training was far more dangerous than the combat missions I participated in.

I learned a great deal and I will share some of it with you. I want to show you how to defend yourself in your own home when an uninvited invader(s) enters your home to do you and your loved ones some serious harm. You have the right to defend yourself.

And you MUST DEFEND yourself & your loved ones or everyone will end up to be another set of DEAD STATISTICS.

⬇
Private Message & Bonus
www.survivalexpertbooks.com/
private-list
(Special Bonus Just For YOU)
⬆

I'll show you some simple tactics that really work that are used by America's military elite units like:
- US Army Delta Force
- US Navy SEALs
- Special A-Teams (Green Berets)
- US Army Rangers
- Special Teams of the US Marine Corps

How can you take-on 01 or more intruders in your home? I'll tell you everything when I send you 03 of these survival tricks FREE!

04) Laydon's Super Quick Burn & Pain Remedy!: Everybody has their own home remedies for this or that. But I will tell you 1st hand:
On 01 Oct. 2006, I stopped the **POUNDING PAIN** after I spilled boiling hot tea directly on my left hand & wrist.

This **super cheap** ingredient worked so good, the **POUNDING PAIN STOPPED** in just 120 seconds flat and never returned and weeks later there were no scars.

It could only happen to me. On 04 Sep. 2015, I was cleaning up my carport. What I didn't know was there was a wasp nest inside a large hose I had hanging up. I reached underneath it and got stung on all 05 fingers of my left hand.

The **PAIN WAS SO AGONIZING** I thought I hit a live wire but there were no live wires.

Like a sissy boy I sprinted to my house and glancing behind me were a few wasps in trail. I went to my medicine cabinet and applied this same cheap ingredient and **IT STOPPED THE POUNDING PAIN IN ALL MY FIVE FINGERS!**

Getting stung 05-times at the same time by multiple wasps would send most people to the hospital. With a co-pay, you're probably out a $100 bucks easy. Not me, I used this super cheap ingredient for just a few bucks. I'm telling you, this super cheap ingredient works so good for STOPPING POUNDING PAIN super quick for:
- Severe burns
- Wasps stings
- Cuts

This super cheap ingredient WORKS SO GOOD it should be in every medicine cabinet, every ambulance, every fire truck, every emergency room, **in your medicine cabinet**,… but it's not.

I have at least 02 of these in my medicine cabinet standing by at all times. And I'll tell you everything once I get your OK to send you your choice of survival tricks!

05) Snakebite & Brown Recluse Spider Bite Remedy!: You don't have to be out in the wilderness to be tagged by venomous snakes. And those venomous Brown Recluse spiders, Black Widow spiders,…are everywhere.

Good folks all over the world purchase my Survival Programs. Many times I talk to folks that are already survival experts in their own right and I am challenged to send them a quality Survival Product.

One day I was talking on the phone to one of my subscribers. Like me, he worked in the jungles of Central America. Initially I thought he was B.S.ing me till he proved himself by saying key things.

Anyway he told me a story of how he learned about a venomous snakebite remedy that is **so effective** it even works **INSTANTLY** for venomous spiders like the Brown Recluse, Black Widow,…

What if you or your loved ones got tagged by a venomous snake or got tagged by a venomous spider and there are NO IMMEDIATE EMERGENCY SERVICES available? You'll know what to do you send me your choice of Survival Tricks.

06) Starting An Emergency Fire - Rub Your Shoe On A Rock!:

I can tell you many true stories where regular folks got in trouble outdoors and froze to death. Some were found with matches on them yet they couldn't start a fire to literally save their lives. I consider myself an expert in emergency fire-starting. Why?

First of all **I DO NOT TEACH** any of the *'rubbing 02 sticks together'* field-craft. Why? Too dang hard to get to work. 2nd, that *'rubbing 02 sticks together'* will NEVER NEVER NEVER NEVER WORK if you're truly hypothermic. Trust me.

Private Message & Bonus
www.survivalexpertbooks.com/
private-list
(Special Bonus Just For YOU)

There's nothing wrong with taking matches and lighters out in the woods with you. But folks have been found DEAD DEAD with matches and lighters on them, yet they couldn't start a fire to literally save their life. I have INVENTED many basic, advanced and ultra-advanced emergency fire-starting applications than you could use on several dozen camping trips.

And one of my many many emergency fire-starting inventions is *Rub Your Shoe On A Rock*. This really works and if you're so hypothermic your hands and fingers will not work. You can't even pull up your zipper or button your coat - your hands and fingers will not work. So using matches and lighters is impossible. And forget about *'rubbing 02 sticks together.'* No bloody way. Using *Rub Your Shoe On A Rock*, you're using the weight of your body to start an emergency fire.

Of all the *8 Elements of Survival* (Fire, Water, Shelter, First-Aid, Signal, Food, Weapons and Navigation) - in my humble opinion, FIRE is the most important in most survival situations. And this unknown fire-starting trick could save your life and those under your care! How does it work? I'll give you all the life-saving details when I send you your choice of Survival Tricks.

07) Panamanian Fishing Trick (100 Fish)!:

Do you like eating breaded fish filets? MMmmmmm! I surely do. This is not a 'fish story.' This is a true story. For about 05-years, back in the 1980s and early 1990s I was stationed at Fort Davis, Panama with a battalion of Army Special Forces (Green Berets) soldiers.

On very rare occasions when the entire battalion was together, we'd have a fish fry. We're talking about 18 A-Teams plus Headquarters company (200+), that's a lot of hungry soldiers.

Where in the heck are they going to get all the fish to feed all these hungry soldiers? I didn't care where the fish came from, I was hungry. Man those breaded fish filets were very very tasty.

Well the years I was down there, I kept hearing the same story of these 02 soldiers from Headquarters Company going out on a boat to Gatun Lake (supports the Panama Canal) and between 7am and about 12 noon, those 02 soldiers would **ALWAYS ALWAYS CATCH ABOUT 100 BASS FISH - GUARANTEED!**

'No way' I thought, it's B.S.

Well towards the end of my tour (July 1991), I decided to track down those 02 soldiers and find out how they were catching 100 bass fish in just 04 hours or so.

Well I tracked them down and they told me exactly what they were LEGALLY doing to catch 100 bass fish (no fish limit in Panama).

Days later I tried it myself just off the bank on Gatun Lake and **BAMM!**

In just a couple minutes, I got me a tasty bass fish real quick. I named this fishing trick - the *Panamanian Fishing Trick*. <u>How does it work?</u> And I'll tell you everything once I get your OK to send you your choice of FREE Survival Tricks.

08) 100% Accurate Weather Forecasting Trick!: Here's a stone cold fact – Mother Nature and all She possesses is the MOST POWERFUL FORCE on Earth. More powerful than all the nukes ever built. And one of the wraths of Mother Nature is weather. I'm going to send you a weather forecasting trick that is 100% accurate! You gotta know when a storm is heading your way. Storms of all sorts hurt & kill people all across the globe <u>EVERY MINUTE OF THE DAY</u>!!! You can use this weather forecasting trick in the woods or even in the city in just 02-seconds. <u>How does it work?</u> I'll tell you everything with your permission to send you any 03 survival tricks.

09) Goose Final Approach!: I use to work at a US government site that required me to have a **TOP SECRET** Security Clearance. It took me a year and a half to get it but I got it. One day while working there, I was talking to one of the janitors. We were talking about hunting and he told me his friend would catch geese without any hunting at all. The geese would fly to him and he'd put that critter on the dinner table. He didn't believe him so his friend invited him out to his house out in the country. Not long after he arrived at his friend's house - **BAMM!** Another goose for the dinner table. When he told me this story, I was amazed but thought - '*talk about thinking outside the box.*' I named this 'no hunting trick' - *Goose Final Approach*.

Private Message & Bonus
www.survivalexpertbooks.com/
private-list
(Special Bonus Just For YOU)

Even World Class hunters don't know about this ingenious 'no hunting trick.' I asked him what about ducks. It's works on ducks too? He didn't know. So here's '*No Weapon Duck Hunting.*'

10) No Weapon Duck Hunting!: I don't know if you've ever tasted duck – it's DELICIOUS! Tastier than chicken, tuna, angus beef, all beef hot dogs,… Here's a real neat survival trick to catch all the ducks you can eat. And I'll explain why it works. I call it '*No Weapon Duck Hunting.*' You:
- Don't need a shotgun
- Don't need a Bola
- Don't need a Duck Call
- Don't need a Trap
- Don't need a Blind

I'll tell you everything once you give me your permission to send you your choice of international survival tricks at absolutely NO-CHARGE.

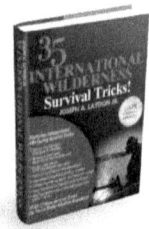
The title of this book is "*35 International Wilderness Survival Tricks!*" – but there are actually 100+ Survival Tricks included in this Survival Book!

I don't advertise the actual number of survival tricks. Only to YOU, a potential customer. And when **YOU PICK YOUR CHOICE OF ANY 03 SURVIVAL TRICKS**, you'll get a good taste of all 100+ survival tricks in this Survival Book. And it's just 01 of my **80+ Survival Books** (Paperback Books & Kindle E-Books – I'm the original writer – no ghost writers).

Included is a website page. It tells you that I'm a real person and I'll send you your choice of survival tricks – FREE at NO CHARGE! PLUS, <u>I HAVE A BONUS WAITING FOR YOU!</u> So go ahead and:
- Go to the website page listed above
- See '*About The Author*'
- Send in Order Form today (next two pages after Testimonials)

Here are couple Testimonials before you fill-out the FREE Order Forms.

Testimonials!

I thought you might like to know what a few of my customers think about my Survival Products. So here are a couple testimonials from a some of my many testimonials.

This first testimonial is from South Africa. This married couple purchased the Flag Ship of my Survival Products, the 60-pound *2012 Ultra-Advanced Anytime Anywhere Survival Program TOTAL Package (2012 U-AASPTP)*. Some of my subscribers are already survival experts in their own right and in this case, this couple ventures into the African wilderness where they are already in the food-chain. There are NO sissy white-tailed deer over there. They are both highly educated (Wallace has a Ph.D. - Doctorate) and both are survival experts in the African wilderness. It was a challenge for me to put a quality Survival Product in front of these 'African survival experts.'

*"Joseph, I can make fire in at least 40 ways. However, you have managed to learn an old dog some new tricks. Joseph, the subjects covered in your news letters, is extremely interesting, researched in depth, and very relevant to the subject of survival, **it stimulates the reader to think lateral**. Joseph, I am impressed with the time and effort you have put into the practical side of your survival program.*

*There are very few view people who actually test things before they publish it, especially to the extent you do I can't stop reading, every day something new is added to my knowledge. Joseph, I have them all (the books, courses, videos and kits), it's my passion survival and bush skills. **Your program... has proven practical information – THE BEST OF THEM ALL – FOR SURE.**"*
                    Wallace V. – South Africa – 15 May 2006

This second testimonial is from a wise subscriber. When I first read the testimonial, I chuckled. But when I re-read it several more times, I finally understood what Richard was really telling me. It's a GREAT COMPLIMENT & TESTIMONIAL from Richard.

*"Your organization was exemplary. **This is indeed the best course I have ever spent any money on, and I have bought many.** If this material was taught to all military personal we would be unstoppable. **RAMBO WISHES HE HAD YOU AS A TEACHER.** Your newsletters let me feel like I am in class, even while on a train, plain, or bus. Your videos are the next best thing if one is not physically there. Every American needs to know this material."*
Richard L. E., Boston - 06 Sep. 2001

Note: Even though Rambo is a bad ass fictional character, do you see what he's trying to say about the Rambo comment?

And this third Testimonial is from Scott, and it is blunt and to the point and compares my Survival Programs against the other Survival books, courses, programs,…. out there. See *"About The Author."*

*"Yes, simply outstanding. This really is a Total Package – professional. **The problem with other programs is amatures training amatures = amatures.** Not so with the Anytime Anywhere Survival Program TOTAL Package (AASPTP). If you want to get past the fantasy & Walter Mitty crap & learn the real life down & dirty survival info **this one is it** (U-AAASPTP). **The survival & fire starting tricks is priceless."***
Scott H., Oklahoma – 24 Jan. 2001

For more Testimonials see www.suvivalexpertbooks.com

Private Mailing List - Order Form - A!

THANK YOU for your very wise interest in my survival work. I promise you I'll give you more than you expect. You'll surely get your money's worth.

My long time philosophy when it comes to teaching international survival is that you're learning from the **REAL SURVIVORS** throughout the globe and throughout history. Here's a partial list of the **REAL SURVIVORS** at www.survivalexpertbooks.com (see *The Real Survivors*)

To send you your choice of Survival Tricks described on the previous pages, I need your permission.

Simply mark (**X**) your choice of Survival Tricks. Before you mark your choices, did you go to **www.survivalexpertbooks.com/private-list?** <u>**I have a BONUS waiting for you!!**</u>

01) _____ PRSC		06) _____ Emergency Fire-Starting…
02) _____ Sauna In A Can		07) _____ Panamanian Fishing…
03) _____ Home Invasion Defense		08) _____ 100% Weather Forecaster
04) _____ Laydon's Burn/Pain Remedy…		09) _____ Goose Final Approach
05) _____ Snakebite/Spider Remedy…		10) _____ No Weapon Duck Hunting

<u>This is **NOT** an E-Mail offer</u>. I will send everything as promised via the good ol' United States Post Service. And I'll send everything via First Class Mail.

Again, this is a **FREE OFFER**. I will send you your choice of Survival Tricks and I WON'T HOLD BACK! You'll get every single word – the full complete details & sketches.

Why am I doing this? I hope to gain your trust so I can send you *"35 International Survival Tricks"* (really 100+ Survival Tricks) for the price of fast food meal.

And even if you decide not to get *"35 International Survival Tricks"*, I'm very confident the Survival Tricks you pick out today will greatly enhance your self-reliance so You're Ready Anytime Anywhere for decades in the future.

NO, I'm not sending you some crap info. In my humble opinion, your choice of Survival Tricks are very worthy of your attention. I'll send EVERYTHING, FREE, as advertised.

To get your choice of Survival Tricks, all you have to do is mark (**X**) your choices above, fill-out the Order Form (both pages) and send them to me. **DO NOT** send me any money. Like I've stated multiple times, this is a **FREE OFFER** to introduce you to my survival work starting in September 1991 to the present day (**www.survivalexpert.com**).

Private Mailing List - Order Form - B!

Fill-out the Order Form below and send it back to me.
I'll get your Survival Tricks in the mail real quick.
I'll send them to you via First Class Mail.

YES Joseph, send me my choice of Survival Tricks. I
understand there is **NO CHARGE** for the Survival Tricks.
I'm sending this Order Form to you today.

_____

PRINT Last Name   First   MI / Jr. Sn.

_____

Street Address / P.O. Box   Apt.

_____

City   State   Zip Code

_____

YOUR SIGNATURE   <u>I AM 21+ Years Of Age</u> Or 17+ (Active Duty USA Military and
Allies). I understand these Survival Tricks are **'For Information Use Only.'** I understand I will
keep this information confidential and will not share this information. I understand this
Survival Information is protected under Unites States of America Copyright Laws.

SEND Order Form Pages To:
Joseph A. Laydon Jr. (IRISAP)
P.O. Box 48
Cutler, IL 62238-0048
United States of America